Grill Cookbo

for Beginners

Easy Grilling Recipes for You to Try and Enjoy With Your Friends and Family

ALBION HOYLES

Table of Contents

Introduction

Grilling meets a range of primitive desires; what is not to appreciate about the T-bone, softly crispy from the outside & tender, juicy, and pink in the middle? It's no joke that grilling is America's favorite pastime because of the unrivaled taste it imparts to beef, seafood, and vegetables.

Everybody, everywhere these days, has a favorite grilling method, custom barbecue, or cookbook, but the final outcome is most often the same: moist, smoky, tasty vegetables and meat grilled on an open fire. The act of lighting a barbecue brings us to our past, encourages us to appreciate the outdoors, and reunites us with the inner cavemen. You do not need a device or high-end rig for the perfect backyard Barbecue this summer; all you need is a basic grill, some beef, & a couple of tricks up the sleeve.

What dilemma is this approach supposed to solve in the kitchen?

We'd have to cook having less heat & lose flavor if we didn't have the grill's searing, intense heat. Caramelization occurs as proteins & sugars experience a transition due to the reaction of Maillard, a chemical process that causes food to be brown when it cooks. This gives grilled vegetables and meat a delightful increase in scent and taste. Consider marshmallows, browned onions, and, of course, the steak.

What exactly is grilling?

Grilling is a dry heat processing technique that uses clear, radiant heat. Grilling helps you to grill vegetables and meat in a limited period of time, which is perfect for every night of every week.

Cooking on such a grill uses a method known as thermal radiation. The heating element may be below or above what is being grilled, and when it's above the beef, it's commonly referred to as "broiled." The majority of grills get their heat from underneath.

Grilling's Advantages

1. Less Body Fat

Less fat is among the most important health effects of grilling. Surplus fat from inside foods drips off before ever reaching the plate, requiring less fat to grill vegetables and meat to perfection. For extra taste and convenience of cooking, mix grilled vegetables in some good olive oil, and a thin coating of a cooking spray can prevent many foods from sticking.

2. Many Nutritious vegetables

Since grilling vegetables requires minimum time than frying them in a conventional oven, they maintain more of the natural nutrients. In the boiling broth, stewed or boiled vegetables lose most of the flavor and also their mineral and vitamin content. Roasted vegetables, on the other hand, keep their shape and color while gaining flavor and nutrients.

3. Meats High in Nutrients

Grilled vegetables are not the only item that becomes more nutritious when grilled over the grill. The riboflavin & thiamine content of meat grilled on the grill is higher. B vitamins such as thiamine & riboflavin help your body convert food into energy. Grilled meat or fish that is thoroughly cooked and not burnt over a flame of gas is an excellent complement to a healthier diet.

4. Cooking with less butter

Meats cooked on a direct heat hold more moisture than meats processed in many other ways. This means the grill master would not be likely to be added more butter to keep the meat juicy when frying. If you use less butter on your meat, you'll get fewer fats on your plate.

5. Grilling is a fun way to spend time with friends and family.

Grilling will improve your morale as well as your physical health. In summers, grilling is a common social activity that allows people to entertain their guests. When tending to the grill, sitting outdoors with friends makes for opportunities for conversation & togetherness, which is beneficial for both your body & mind.

Kinds of charcoal: Lump vs. Briquettes

Using charcoal to light a fire in a grill

Lump charcoal burns hotter than the briquettes, although it can take some care to maintain a constant temperature. Briquettes, not like pure charcoal, are compressed wood by-products with additives & chemicals to make them light easily and flame evenly. They have a more continuous burn than lump charcoal, keeping a sustained temperature for such a long period and less hand-holding. Briquettes may be lit with a cigarette, whereas lump charcoal involves the use of the chimney starter and lighter fluid. The following directions will teach you how to burn lump charcoal in two separate ways.

What is the best way to light a barbecue grill?

Charcoal is being lit.

To light charcoal with a chimney starter, follow these steps:

A chimney booster, a metallic cylinder including a handle which makes the lighting coals a breeze, is maybe the best way to ignite the charcoal grill of all.

1. Filled your chimney having the necessary volume of charcoal & put it over the grill's bottom grate. A typical chimney holds around 100 briquets, yet depending on the scale of your chimney, you do not need as many.

2. Check the directions on your chimney to add either one or around two layers of newspaper on the base of your starter. Several spots in the newspaper should be lit. The fires from the burning newspaper inside the chamber beneath light the outlines of your charcoal above. Check the chimney vents to see if your coals have begun to burn and the sides of the coals are in grey.

3. After 8 to 10 minutes, you can see that the coals are glowing via the vents & flames flickering on the upper layer of the coals. Wait until you see the coals get mostly coated in ash & gray in color before pouring them in a pile. The coals could then be scattered out. It takes about 15 minutes to complete the process.

How to light charcoal with lighter fluid

1. If you've got the chimney starter, this can completely eliminate the use of lighter fluid, resulting in a cleaner flavor and fewer additives. If you've no option but to do the lighter fluid, always use it cautiously and according to the instructions on the label.

2. Place the charcoal in the middle of the grill's bottom grate.

3. Immediately squirt the lighter fluid over the light and coals. Never squirt the liquid into hot coals that are ignited or smoking.

4. When the coals are coated with gray ash, they are good to use.

Grilling with wood

1. Wood chips in a barbecue's smoker tray

2. Try grilling on an open flame or with wood chips if you are able to move the grilling game to the next level. It's not for the novice griller because you'll need a secure place for the fire pit and the grill, which can handle a natural wood fire, which can be pricey. The flavor is simple outdoors, just the person and the beef, with a little additional smoke thrown in for good measure.

3. Hardwoods such as pecan, oak, maple, alder, hickory or beech should be seasoned (dried). Softwoods, such as fir and pine, release a cloud of smoke which destroys the taste of the food.

4. You could be aware of the following steps if you've ever created a campfire and ignited a flame in a fireplace: Build a teepee out of tiny twigs on top of the pile of firewood (newspaper, tinder and wood chips), and add bigger bits of wood while the fire gets going. The chimney starter may also be used to light a wood fire. Cover your chimney with chunks of hardwood and light it like a fireplace. Alternatively, ignite any charcoal inside your chimney starter under fire to help the wood catch fire.

5. Allow your fire to grow & burn it down to flames for up to around 45 minutes. Then scrape the blazing orange flames under your grill grate with such a shovel or the long grill hoe handle. The high your heat, just as with the charcoal, the deep the mound. Cooking over surging flames is a widespread misunderstanding among newcomers to wood fire cooking.

6. Neither lump charcoal nor charcoal briquettes burn as quickly as wood. Make sure the embers are replenished every 20-30 minutes.

7. Many states ban open fires, such as those constructed on the floor or inside a pit. Before you start grilling, make sure to check with the local authority. If you'd like to try grilling with wood, an indoor fireplace wood burning is too an option.

To cedar the plank or not, that is the issue.

In a grill, salmon is served on a wood plank.

1. Cooking the food directly over the plank, a few of the small boards offered by the box in the section of grilling inside the supermarkets, entails cooking the food on the bit of wood. The aim of using the cedar plank is just to impart some of the wood's flavor to your food. Not just you decide which form of wood will fit well with the food you're grilling, and you must also ensure that it won't burn while you're doing so.

2. Choose ash or cedar for fragile foods like tuna. We've fried salmon on cedar planks before. For bolder meats such as pork or chicken, apple, maple or pecan are fine options, while hickory, mesquite or oak can stick the strong tastes of lamb, game or beef.

3. Soak a plank in cold water for at least 1 hour before using it to enable that water to soak in the wood. Working just over the indirect aspect of the two-zone fire is the most popular cooking process. This will ensure slow, steady, gentle heat during the cooking process, enabling you to spend a lot of time mostly on the grill & allowing flavors to marry and mingle. Using this approach, you would be allowed to reuse the planks sometimes.

4. The second approach entails charring the plank first on the hot part of your grill, then shifting it over the cooler part and putting the food over it. This method can enhance the smokiness of the meat.

Cleaning, lubricating, & maintaining the grills are all necessary.

Cleaning your latches of the barbecue with a bit of wood

Cleaning the grill at the start of the grilling session, when the grill is heating up, is the most effective method. It is simple to get your fire to do the rest of the job. Preheating the grill for around ten minutes and even more than that is enough time for burning your food from the previous cooking session. You may also drive over the grates with the edge of the pair of the long tongs, the grill brush, or even the grill brick. To prepare the grates for cooking pizzas, vegetables, or beef, dip your paper towel inside a few neutral cooking oils & roll it across the grates using your tongs.

Enable it to cool before gently brushing the grates using a brush of grill after you've done grilling. Before storing the barbecue, clean it off with a rag, empty the ashes, & close it. Allowing rain to enter the grill & corrode the inside is not a good idea.

Achieving Ideal Grill Marks

1. On the oven, a nice fried chicken breast

2. The cross-hatching picture-perfect of a finely grilled chicken chop or breast is maybe the best aspect of grilling. Here's how to really get great scores.

3. To ensure your grill is nice & hot, preheat it for around 10 to 15 minutes.

4. Before grilling, brush the meat with a thin layer of grease.

5. Place the meat on the grill grates and sear it. When the meat is finished, it will detach, but if you're not positive, you can test it with the edge of a spatula. It's definitely not ready if your meat holds together. Return it to its original position and wait.

6. To have your grill mark's X, turn your meat at about an angle of 45-degree. The middle axis point should be the middle of whatever you're grilling. Wait before the meat escapes spontaneously through the grates before flipping, but it shouldn't take a longer time than before.

7. You can only be concerned about making one side of your vegetables or meat seared perfectly; else, you may risk overcooking.

When it comes to heat, there are two types: indirect and direct.

Under the grilling grates of a barbecue, there are hot coals.

Obviously, the purpose of grilling should be to achieve a wonderfully seared slab of meat; however, there are some tricks to using the grill to have both direct & indirect heat areas, which is essential for cooking bigger sections such as roasts or chickens despite burning them. Variable zones on gas grills may help achieve a reasonable indirect/direct balance, so each grill is special. Building those areas on a barbecue grill, on the other hand, is totally up to ourselves:

Direct fire: For pretty hot, one-zone grilling, this setup uses coals dispersed uniformly at the base of a grill. It is a nice setup for vast volumes of food, such as steaks & burgers.

Two main direct fire: This configuration holds the burning coals with one side of your grill with just a few on the other to keep the food warm. This method works well for chicken and other foods which need a strong sear, mostly on the warm side followed by the indirect heat for finish cooking.

In a two-zone indirect fire, all of the charcoal is filled on 1 side while the other is left bare. This is a great way to serve roasts & whole chickens.

Coals are piled against both the edges of your grill in the three-zone split burn, making a section of your grill vacant down the center. For the pork roasts & smaller roasts, use this method.

Keeping an eye on the temperature of the grill

A barbecue's temperature gauge is located on the cover.

When do you protect with a cap, and when do you leave it open?

Although it is tempting to check the beef, when should the grill be left open and when should it be closed? This is a simple one. Keep your lid off if the food you're preparing is 3/4" or more thinner, such as tiny asparagus or zucchini strips. Shut the lid while you're frying pork chops thickly cut, corn over the cob, and chicken breasts. By closing the door, you can take a maximum of the grill's well-known convection fire.

How to adjust your grill's vents

Last but not least, most of the charcoal grills include vents over both the top and bottom sides. When they are free, the warm air within the grill exits via the top, producing a negative air region that pulls colder air in thru the lower vent. The new oxygen which is pulled in assists in preserving the fire's heat. In reality, the grill with the open vents burns hotter or one with closed vents. Try shutting the vents if you want to keep it cold.

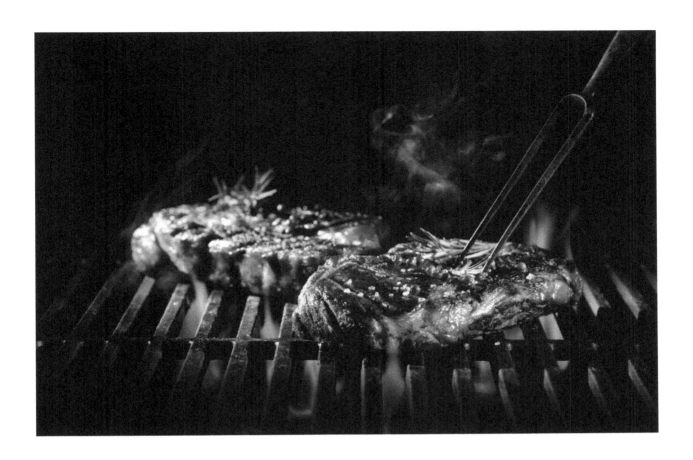

Chapter 1: Grilling Basics

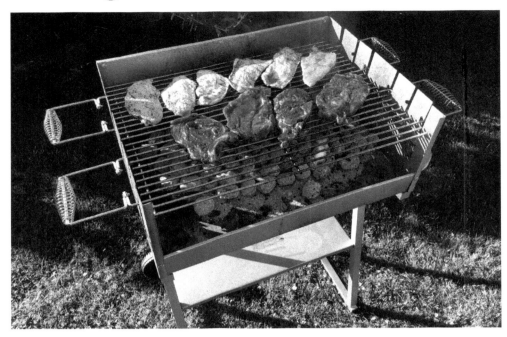

1.1 Grilling tips and techniques

There are a range of grilling styles and approaches to pick from. There are several different kinds of sources of heat for grilling. When you consider the various forms of food available, such as steaks, chicken, fish, shrimp, and vegetables, it's easy to see how grilling can be accomplished in a number of ways.

The trick is to tailor the grilling techniques & equipment to the type of food you're grilling in order to achieve the desired outcome. These considerations must be weighed in order to achieve the best outcomes from a given approach or procedure.

Food form, heat source, & desired outcome are the most important considerations. The final consideration is a personal choice or temperature; as in, can you barbecue indoors or outside?

Methods of Grilling

Grilling having direct heat is by far the most simple and widely used way of grilling. This method's words say for themselves. To cook food, it is put directly on the heat source. On can do this on gas, charcoal, wood or some other form of the heat source.

The temperature is normally very high, which is perfect for searing. To seal tastes, searing means using a high amount of heat to 'cook' all sides of the item of food for just several minutes. The longer one can sear the meat, the thicker it is.

Outdoor Grills with a Flaming

After searing, your food can be shifted to the 'not really hot' portion of your grill to finish cooking.

Direct heat is ideal for hamburgers, steaks, ribs, sausages, and even kabobs. Cooking time for these ingredients is typically 30 minutes or less.

Indirect grilling, known as a cooking technique that uses indirect or reflected heat to cook the food.

It means not cooking the food directly over a heat source & having the lid closed for the rest of the period.

If your food has to be put over a heat source, the temperature must be kept low enough that the food can cook 'indirectly.' This is similar to roasting in the oven. This method can be used to cook large parts which take a long time to cook, such as the leg of the lamb, whole turkeys and several roasts.

Food products are often grilled over overt heat at first to lock in flavors before being cooked over indirect heat.

One of the grilling methods that involve a more advanced approach is smoking. It's just possible to do it outside. While grilling using gas or charcoal, you can smoke your food. The actual procedure entails boiling food at such a low temperature in such a sealed chamber for a prolonged period of time, hence the word 'low & slow in the industry.

To 'flavor' the meal, use some of the favorite hardwood smoking chips of wood, pellets, chunks or even ashes. That heat source normally occurs near your food or sometimes in a separate chamber or crate.

The end product is normally moist, smoky food. You must know what we are talking about. For the serious smoker,' special equipment is required.

One of the most common grilling methods is rotisserie grilling. Spit roasting is another name for it. Food is put in a compartment with a spinning skewer or a motorized spin spit in this form. Now, indirect heat required for cooking is generated by special ceramic and infrared burners. Indirect heat can sometimes be produced using charcoal fire.

A motor assembly already builds in some new grills rotates the beef. If the grill doesn't have one, after-market engines are eligible for 'learn it yourself. This technique can be used to cook entire chickens, roasts, & ribs.

Grilling Food Outside in the Summer

Outdoor grilling isn't really a grilling process in and of itself.

It merely applies to the act of cooking outside. To learn more, look up charcoal, petrol, or wood grilling.

Grilling with planks is a one-of-a-kind activity.

The concept is to put food over a bit of wood, which smolder-smoke' & infuse your foodstuff with the wood flavor as the heat is applied.

Planks are easily available for purchase on the internet. Cedar planks, as well as other different wood planks, can be sold in the most reliable retail gourmet & grilling equipment shops. Call out your own spice planks if you can't spot them. Just kidding.

Infrared grilling has been a little grilling process. No one in the world is sure of it. That'd be the weirdest day of your life, wouldn't it? Infrared is a heat-generating process that is both 'low-tech' & 'high-tech.'

On the one hand, one industry insider compares infrared heat with the heat generated by a bonfire that travels to the face by heat waves rather than wind. Isn't it a little low-tech?

On the other side, we realize that new ceramic infrared grilling burners are built to produce incredibly high heat, so this is hi-tech. All of the fat has disappeared! Infrared grills are more expensive. It's been heard that their rates are coming down. Applying infrared heat in grilling has both advantages and drawbacks.

Grilling Methods

The most common and popular method of grilling is with charcoal. It is very flexible and covers all facets of grilling. Charcoal briquettes or lump charcoal are used as food.

To render wonderful grilled meats, both indirect and direct grilling heat methods & techniques may be used. Furthermore, charcoal grills seem very cheap and can be sold in many retail and hardware stores.

There's a slew of grilling advice at your fingertips.

There is still a lively discussion over whether to use charcoal or gas. Which alternative do you choose?

Grilling with gas is known to be the most efficient method of cooking. It's a 'no-mess grilling process. Gas grills are usually more costly than charcoal grills, but they compensate for it by being quite compact, and temperature regulation is a breeze.

It's much easier to fire a gas grill, and there's no smoke.' There will be some assembly needed. Carefully observe the assembly directions. After that, all you'll need is a portable tank loaded with liquid propane, natural gas, and any other permitted petroleum gas available in the region. The gas grill becomes quick to use after it has been fitted up.

Wood grilling, a method of grilling that uses wood as a fuel source. Until recently, this form of grilling has only been found in restaurants. For house cooking, there are heavy-duty, compact grills of wood-burning and stoves on the marketplace currently.

Wood burns more easily than charcoal, so this imparts rich flavors of oak, hickory, as well as other citrus woods, including cherry. Aged log, which has been cut down and frozen for at least a year before use, burns more efficiently and produces less smoke in the stove.

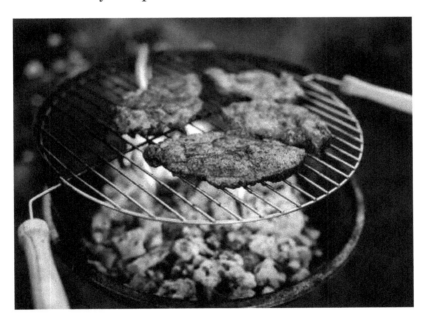

Chapter 2: Grill Breakfast Recipes

1. Scrambled eggs (cast-iron)

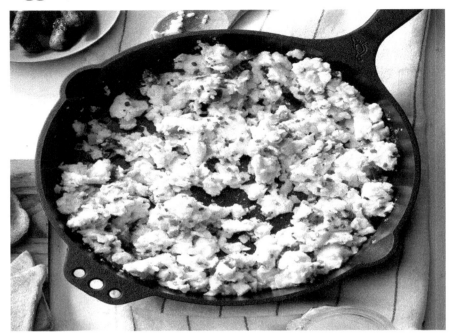

Cook Time: 25 Minutes

Serving: 6 people

Difficulty: Easy

Ingredients:

- 1 seeded & chopped jalapeno pepper

- 12 big eggs

- 3 tbsp. minced chives

- 1/4 tsp. pepper

- 1/4 tsp. salt

- 2/3 cup sweet onion finely chopped

- 1 log (four ounces) fresh goat crumbled cheese

Instructions:

1. In a big bowl, beat the eggs, pepper and salt, water and set aside.

2. Preheat the grill rack to medium-high heat and place a 10-inch cast-iron pan on it. Cook onion & jalapeno with butter in a pan until tender. Cook, stirring continuously until the egg mixture is nearly set. Cook & stir until the eggs are fully set, and then add the cheese & chives.

2. Prosciutto Panini egg

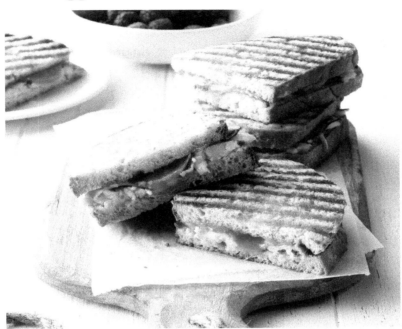

Cook Time: 4 minutes

Serving: 8

Difficulty: Easy

Ingredients:

- 3 big eggs

- 2 big egg whites

- 6 tbsp. milk (fat-free)

- 1 thinly sliced green onion

- 1 tbsp. Dijon mustard

- 1 tbsp. maple syrup

- 8 slices of sourdough bread

- 8 thin slices deli ham of prosciutto

- 1/2 cup of cheddar cheese, shredded sharp

- 8 tsp. butter

Instructions:

1. In a shallow dish, mix the eggs, onion, milk and egg whites. Place a big skillet over medium heat and coat it with cooking spray. Cook & stir the egg mixture on medium heat till it is fully formed.

2. Combine the mustard and the syrup and spread it on four slices of bread. Scrambled eggs, cheese and prosciutto, are layered on top of the leftover bread. Sandwiches should have butter on the outside.

3. Cook for around 3 to 4 minutes on an indoor grill or the panini maker, or till bread becomes browned & cheese gets melted. To eat, cut every panini in half.

3. Foil-Packet sausage and potatoes

Cook Time: 30 minutes

Serving: 8 people

Difficulty: Easy

Ingredients:

- 3 pounds of red potatoes sliced into cubes of 1/2-inch

- 2 packages (i.e., every 12 ounces) sausage links, sliced into slices of 1/2-inch

- 4 cooked & crumbled bacon strips

- 1 chopped medium onion

- 2 tbsp. of fresh parsley, chopped

- 1/4 tsp. salt

- 1/4 tsp. garlic salt

- 1/4 tsp. pepper

- Additional fresh parsley, chopped (optional)

Instructions:

1. Prepare a medium-heat grill or medium heat. Toss potatoes including sausage, parsley, pepper, onion, bacon and salts in a big mixing cup.

2. Cover eight 18x12-inch squares of high-duty foil that is nonstick with the paste, putting food on the bland side of the foil. Fold the foil securely over the potato mixture to cover it.

3. Cook for around 15 minutes on either side or till potatoes become tender over a grill or campfire. Carefully open the packets to enable steam to pass. Additional parsley may be added if needed.

4. Grilled Ginger-Glazed Honeydew

Cook Time: 5 minutes

Serving: 6 people

Difficulty: Easy

Ingredients:

- 1/4 cup of peach preserves

- 1 tbsp. lemon juice

- 1 tbsp. crystallized ginger, finely chopped

- 2 tsp. of lemon zest, grated

- 1/8 tsp. of ground cloves

- 1 honeydew melon of medium size, sliced into cubes of 2-inch

Instructions:

1. Combine peaches, lemon juice, ginger and clove in a shallow cup. Brush half of the glaze onto six metal or coated wooden skewers with honeydew.

2. Grill honeydew on a finely oiled rack over a moderate flame, sealed, for around 4 to 6 minutes, rotating and basting regularly with leftover glaze, or griddle 4 in. from heat, only before melon starts to soften & brown.

5. Éclairs over the grill

Cook Time: 5 minutes

Serving: 6 people

Difficulty: Easy

Ingredients:

- 1/2 cup of chocolate frosting

- Whipped cream

- Wooden or stick dowel (length: 24 inches and diameter 5/8 inch)

- 3 cups of chocolate or vanilla pudding (snack size)

- 1 tube refrigerated smooth dough sheet (eight ounces)

Instructions:

1. Prepare a high-heat grill or campfire. Wrap foil around one of the ends of the wooden dowel or stick. Break the crescent dough into 6 4-inch squares after unrolling it. Wrap the single piece of dough all around the ready stick, pinching the end & seam together to seal it.

2. Cook for 5-7 minutes over a grill or campfire, turning regularly until it gets golden brown. Remove dough from stick until it is cool to touch. Allow cooling completely. Repeat for the remainder of the dough.

3. Make a tiny hole in one side of a sealed plastic bag and place the pudding inside. To press the mixture inside each shell, squeeze the bag. Cover it with the whipped cream and a layer of frosting.

6. Campfire Hash

Cook Time: 40 minutes

Serving: 6 people

Difficulty: Easy

Ingredients:

- 1 large chopped onion

- 2 tbsp. canola oil

- 2 minced garlic cloves

- 4 cubed and peeled large potatoes (around 2 pounds)

- 1 pound sliced and halved polish sausage or smoked kielbasa

- 1 can green chilies chopped (4 ounces)

- 1 can drain full kernel corn (around 15-1/4 ounces)

Instructions:

1. Cook & stir onion in the oil in a big ovenproof skillet in medium heat until tender. Cook for an additional minute after adding the garlic. Toss in the peas. Cook for around 20 minutes, uncovered, stirring regularly.

2. After adding kielbasa, cook, occasionally stirring, until the meat & potatoes are tender & browned around 10-15 minutes. The heat from the chiles and maize.

7. Breakfast Burger

Cook Time: 30 minutes

Serving: 4 people

Difficulty: Easy

Ingredients:

- 1 pound of ground beef

- 1 tbsp. Worcestershire sauce

- 1 tsp. Montreal seasoning steak

- 1/2 tsp. salt, divided

- 1/2 tsp. pepper, divided

- 3 tbsp. butter, softened & divided

- 8 slices of Texas toast

- 2 tbsp. of canola oil

- 2-1/2 cups of harsh brown frozen shredded potatoes, thawed

- 4 big eggs

- 1/4 cup of spreadable fruit seedless blackberry

- 4 slices of American cheese

- 8 bacon strips, cooked

Instructions:

1. Lightly and thoroughly add Worcestershire sauce, grounded beef, 1/4 tsp. Salt, 1/4 tsp. of pepper and steak seasoning. Form four 1/2-inch-thick patties. Cover and cook burgers on an oiled grill rack on medium heat for 4-5 minutes on either side till a thermometer gets on160°.

2. In the meantime, sprinkle 2 tbsp. Butter on one side of the slices of Texas toast and grill with the burgers once golden brown. Remove the burgers & toast from the heat and set them aside to stay warm.

3. Turn on the heat to heavy. Heat the oil in a big skillet on the grill rack. With 1/2 cupfuls, put hash browns into oil and press to compress. Add the remaining salt & pepper to taste. Fry, sealed, for around 12 to 15 minutes on every hand, till golden brown & crisp, including oil as required. Remove from the oven and stay warm.

4. Reduce to a medium heat environment. Heat the leftover butter in the same pan. Fry the eggs over the low sun.

5. To assemble, spread 4 Texas toast slices with blackberry spread. 1 patty of hash brown color, 2 strips of bacon, 1 egg fried, 1 burger, 1 slice of cheese are layered on every slice. Add the remaining slices of toast on top.

8. Packet and cheesy ham

Cook Time: 20 minutes

Serving: 4 people

Difficulty: Easy

Ingredients:

- 1-1/2 pounds red medium potatoes, thinly sliced and halved

- 1 medium chopped green pepper

- 1 medium chopped onion

- 1/4 tsp. pepper

- 2 cups of deli ham, cubed

- 1 cup cheddar cheese, shredded

Instructions:

1. Mix potatoes with onion, pepper and green pepper in a big mixing bowl; put in the middle of an oiled 24x18-in. The sheet of high-duty foil. To seal the veggies, fold the foil around them and crimp the ends.

2. Cover and grill for around 15 to 20 minutes over a moderate flame or till potatoes are soft. Remove the grill from the heat. Carefully open the foil to allow steam to evaporate. Toss in the ham and cheese. Cover and continue to grill for another 2-4 minutes or till cheese becomes melted.

9. Grilled Fruits stone with the Balsamic Syrup

Cook Time: 8 minutes

Serving: 4 people

Difficulty: Easy

Ingredients:

- 1/2 cup of balsamic vinegar

- 2 tbsp. brown sugar

- 2 peeled & halved medium peaches

- 2 peeled & halved medium nectarines

- 2 peeled & halved medium plums

Instructions:

1. Combine vinegar & brown sugar in a shallow saucepan. Bring it to a boil, and then simmer until the liquid has been reduced significantly.

2. Grill peaches, plums and nectarines covered on a finely greased grill rack over the moderate flame or griddle 4 in. from heat once soft, 3 to 4 minutes along both sides.

3. Fruits should be diced and put on a serving tray. Drizzle the sauce on top.

10. Breakfast Skewers

Cook Time: 8 minutes

Serving: 5 people

Difficulty: Easy

Ingredients:

- 1 package (around 7 ounces) frozen breakfast fully cooked thawed sausage links

- 1 can (around 20 ounces) drained pineapple chunks

- 10 fresh mushrooms, medium

- 2 tbsp. butter, melted

- Maple syrup

Instructions:

1. Cut the sausages in equal parts; alternately string sausages, mushrooms and pineapple on 5 metal or coated wooden skewers. Brush with melted butter and maple syrup.

2. Grill for around 8 minutes, alternating & frying with syrup, uncovered, on medium heat, till sausages are gently browned & fruit is cooked through.

11. Grilled zesty ham

Cook Time: 10 minutes

Serving: 4 people

Difficulty: Easy

Ingredients:

- 1/3 cup of brown sugar, packed

- 2 tbsp. prepared horseradish

- 4 tsp. lemon juice

- 1 fully cooked (1 pound) bone ham steak

Instructions:

1. In a shallow saucepan, combine the brown sugar, lemon juice and horseradish; bring it to boil,

stirring continuously. Brush all sides of the ham.

2. Place the ham on a grill rack that has been oiled over moderate flame. Grill, sealed, for 7 to 10 minutes, until it's glazed and cooked through, rotating periodically.

12. Grilled Herb Potatoes

Cook Time: 25 minutes

Serving: 4 people

Difficulty: Easy

Ingredients:

- 1 pound (about 16) small red potatoes, halved

- 1/4 cup of cranberry juice

- 2 tbsp. butter, cubed

- 1 tsp. each rosemary, oregano, thyme and fresh dill (minced)

- 1/2 tsp. salt

- 1/8 tsp. pepper

Instructions:

1. Combine all the ingredients in a big mixing bowl; transfer to a high-duty aluminum foil board (around 18 to 12-in. rectangle). Fold the foil securely over the mixture to secure it.

2. Cover and cook for around 25 to 30 minutes over a moderate flame or till potatoes are soft. Carefully open the foil to enable steam to pass.

13. Blueberry-Cinnamon Campfire Bread

Cook Time: 30nminutes

Serving: 8 people

Difficulty: Easy

Ingredients:

- 1 loaf (about 1 pound) bread, cinnamon-raisin

- 6 big eggs

- 1 cup around 2% of milk or half & half cream

- 2 tbsp. maple syrup

- 1 tsp. vanilla extract

- 1/2 cup of chopped toasted pecans

- 2 cups of divided fresh blueberries

Instructions:

1. Prepare a low-heat grill or campfire. Adjust bread slices into a double sheet of heavy-duty aluminum foil that has been greased (about 24 into18 in.). Wrap the foil across the sides of the plate, making sure that the top accessible. Combine the vanilla, milk, eggs and syrup in a mixing cup. Pour over the bread and top with 1 cup of blueberries and nuts. Fold the top edges over and crimp to cover.

2. Put on your grill grate in a grill or campfires for 30 to 40 minutes or till eggs are fully cooked. Remove it from the heat and set it aside for 10 minutes. Serve with the leftover blueberries and more maple syrup when needed.

14. Egg & Spinach Breakfast Burritos

Cook Time: 30 minutes

Serving: 10 people

Difficulty: Easy

Ingredients:

- 1 pound of bulk lean turkey breakfast sausage

- 1 tbsp. of canola oil

- 1 cup of hash brown frozen cubed potatoes, thawed

- 1 chopped tiny red onion

- 6 cups (around 4 ounces) of coarsely chopped fresh spinach

- 6 big beaten eggs

- 10 multigrain (8 inches) tortillas, warmed

- 3/4 cup of crumbled feta cheese or queso fresco

- Salsa and guacamole, optional

Instructions:

1. Cook sausage in a big skillet over moderate heat until it is no longer pink, around 4 to 6 minutes, splitting it up into crumbles; take it out from the pan.

2. Heat the oil in the same skillet. Cook, occasionally stirring, until potatoes, pepper and onions are soft, around 5 to 7 minutes. Stir in the spinach for 1-2 minutes or until it has wilted. Cook and whisk the sausage and eggs till all the liquid egg

3. Fill each tortilla with 1/2 cup of filling and a sprinkling of cheese. Fold the bottom & sides of the rollover the filling & fold it up. Serve with salsa and guacamole, if needed.

Choice 1: Ice the filling before assembling the burritos. Burritos should be individually wrapped in foil & frozen in a plastic storage freezer container. Freeze for more than a month in the freezer. Thaw partly overnight in the refrigerator/cooler before using. Prepare a medium-heat campfire. Cover foil-wrapped burritos in aluminum foil and put on your grill grate on the grill or campfire. Grill for 25 to 30 minutes, regularly rotating, until thoroughly cooked.

15. Scrambled Egg Bread

Cook Time: 10 minutes

Serving: 4 people

Difficulty: Easy

Ingredients:

• 1 loaf (about 1 pound) of French bread unsliced

• 2 tbsp. of softened butter, divided

Filling:

• 2 tbsp. o butter, divided

• 1 chopped small onion

• 1 cup of fully cubed cooked ham

• 1 chopped large tomato

• 6 big eggs

• 1/8 tsp. pepper

• 1-1/2 cups of shredded divided cheddar cheese

Instructions:

1. Prepare a medium-heat grill or campfire. Cut each slice of bread in half lengthwise and crosswise. Two bits are hollowed out, leaving 1/2-inch shells. Remove the bread and break it into cubes; set aside 1-1/2 cups 1 tbsp. of softened butter, spread on bread shells. Over the remaining bread halves, scatter the remaining softened butter. Delete from the equation.

2. 1 tbsp. Butter warmed over a campfire in a shallow Dutch oven. Cook & stir for 3 to 4 minutes, or until onion is tender. Remove the skillet from the heat and stir in the ham and tomato.

3. Whisk eggs & pepper together in a shallow cup. Heat the remaining butter in the same skillet. Pour in the egg mixture and fry, constantly stirring until the eggs have thickened and no visible egg is left. Combine the ham paste, 1 cup of cheese, and the leftover bread cubes in a mixing dish. Cover bread shells halfway with filling; top with leftover cheese. Cover it with foil and move to a 13 by 9-inch removable foil pan.

4. Place the pan on top of the campfire. Cook for 8 to 10 minutes, or until cheese gets melted and cooked through. Cook saved bread halves for about 1 to 2 minutes, buttered it side down until toasted. Each slice of egg toast should be cut in half and toasted.

16. Dutch Cheesy Oven Bacon and Eggs

Cook Time: 25 minutes

Serving: 8 people

Difficulty: Easy

Ingredients:

- 1 pound of chopped bacon strips

- 1 package (around 20 ounces) refrigerated hash brown O'Brien potatoes

- 8 big eggs

- 1/2 cup of half & half cream

- 1/2 to 1 tsp. of pepper sauce hot, optional

- 2 cups of cheddar-Monterey shredded Jack cheese

Instructions:

1. Make a moderate heat grill or campfire with 32 to 36 of charcoal briquettes or big wood chips.

2. Heat bacon in a 10-inch Dutch oven over a campfire till crisp, stirring periodically. Drain it on the paper towels after removing using a rubber spatula. 2 teaspoons of the drippings should be kept in the tub.

3. Cautiously press potatoes into the bottom of the Dutch oven & 1 inch up the sides. In a shallow cup, whisk together the eggs, milk, and pepper sauce, if using. Pour over the potatoes and finish with fried bacon and shredded cheese.

4. Cover the Dutch oven with a lid. Place the Dutch oven right above 16-18 briquettes when wood chips or briquettes are fully coated in white ash. Position 16 to 18 briquettes onto pan cover with long-handled tongs.

5. Cook for 20 to 25 minutes or till the eggs are fully cooked, and the cheese has melted. To search for doneness, gently raise the cover with tongs. Cook for an additional 5 minutes if possible.

17. Grilled Breakfast Bistro Sandwiches

Cook Time: 30 minutes

Serving: 2 people

Difficulty: Easy

Ingredients:

- 2 tsp. butter, divided
- 4 big eggs, beaten
- 4 slices of (3/4 thick) Italian bread
- 1/8 tsp. of salt
- 1/8 tsp. of pepper
- 4 ounces of smoked cheddar cheese or smoked Gouda, cut into four slices
- 1 medium thinly sliced pear
- 4 cooked slices of Canadian bacon
- 1/2 cup of small fresh spinach

Instructions:

1. In a medium nonstick pan, melt 1 tsp. of butter over moderate heat; Include eggs & scramble till set. Divide the eggs into pieces of bread and season them with pepper and salt on both ends. Pear slices, cheese slices, spinach and Canadian bacon, layered between slices of bread. Finish with the remaining bread.

2. Layer the leftover butter on each side of the sandwiches if you use a panini maker. According to the manufacturer's instructions, grill for about 6 to 8 minutes, or till golden brown & grill marks appear.

3. Place half of the available butter on one side of the sandwiches if you are using the indoor grill. Place the buttered piece down on the grill and weigh it down with such a large skillet or something else. Grill for about 3 to 5 minutes over a moderate flame, or till golden brown & grill-marked. Remove the weight and butter; it's the other part of the sandwiches. Replace the weight and return to the grill, having buttered piece down. Grill for another 3 o t5 minutes, or till golden brown.

Chapter 3: Recipes for Grilled Seafood

1. Shrimp butter on the grill

Cook Time: 9 minutes

Serving: 6 people

Difficulty: Easy

Ingredients:

- 6 tbsp. butter (unsalted)

- 1/2 cup red onion, finely chopped

- 1 1/2 tsp. red pepper, crushed

- 1 tsp. shrimp paste from Malaysia

- 1 1/2 tbsp. lime juice, freshly squeezed

- Black pepper

- Salt

- 24 wide shelled & deveined shrimp

- 6 big wooden skewers, submerged for 30 minutes in water

- For garnish, leaves of torn mint and various sprouts

Instructions:

1. 3 tbsp. butter, melted in a deep skillet. Cook, occasionally stirring, until the onion is softened, around 3 minutes. Cook, stirring continuously, for 2 minutes, until the smashed red pepper & shrimp paste are fragrant. Season with lime juice and salt, as well as the leftover 3 tbsp. of butter. Heat the butter with the shrimp.

2. Preheat the grill or a grill tray. Season your shrimp with pepper and salt before threading those onto the drumsticks (don't overcrowd them). Grill for 4 mins totals over high temperature, rotating once, until finely charred and only cooked through. Transfer to a serving platter and finish with shrimp butter. Serve garnished with sprouts and mint leaves.

2. Corn salad with grilled scallops

Cook Time: 9 minutes

Serving: 6 people

Difficulty: Easy

Ingredients:

- Six ears of barley, peeled and shucked

- 1 pint halved grape tomatoes

- 3 scallions, finely cut white & light green pieces only

- 1/3 cup finely sliced basil leaves

- Season with salt & freshly ground pepper.

- 1 minced tiny shallot

- 2 tbsp. balsamic vinaigrette

- 2 tsp. boiling water

- 1 teaspoon mustard (Dijon)

- 3 tbsp. safflower oil plus 1/4 cup

- a pound and a half of sea scallops (around 30)

Instructions:

1. Cook your corn till soft in a big tub of salted boiling water, around 5 minutes. Drain and set aside to cool. Remove the kernels from the corn and put it in a large. Season it with salt & pepper, and add scallions, tomatoes and basil.

2. Puree your shallot, adding the vinegar, boiling wine, and mustard in a blender. Slowly drizzle in 6 teaspoons of safflower oil while the blender is working. Toss the corn salad with the vinaigrette, seasoning it with pepper and salt.

3. Toss the scallops with the remaining one tbsp. of oil in a big mixing bowl; season with pepper and salt. A big grill pan should be heated. Put 1/2 of your scallops to the pan at one time and cook, rotating once, till browned, around 4 minutes each batch, over medium-high heat. Serve your corn salad piled high on plates with your scallops on top.

3. Honeydew-avocado salad with grilled scallops

Cook Time: 8 minutes

Serving: 4 people

Difficulty: Easy

Ingredients:

- 2 tsp. new lime juice, lime zest finely grated

- 1 tbsp. olive oil extra-virgin, plus a little extra for drizzling

- 1 1/2 cups honeydew melon, crust removed & split into 1/4-inch dice

- 1 avocado, chopped into around 1/4-inch cubes

- Salt and black pepper, newly roasted

- Big sea scallops weighing 2 pounds

Instructions:

1. Preheat the barbecue. Merge juice & lime zest with 1 tbsp. of olive oil inside a big mixing cup. Fold the sliced honeydew melon & avocado with a rubber spatula. Season your salsa with black pepper and salt.

2. Season the scallops with salt & black pepper after drizzling them with olive oil. 3 - 4 minutes each side over medium-high heat, rotating once, till nicely charred & only cooked through. Move your scallops in the plates and serve with the salsa on the side.

4. Seafood grilled kebabs & arugula orecchiette

Cook Time: 12 minutes

Serving: 4 people

Difficulty: Easy

Ingredients:

- 8 super-sized scallops, halved (approximately 2 ounces each)

- 16 big shelled & deveined shrimp (about 1 pound)

- A dozen cherry tomatoes

- Season with salt & freshly ground pepper.

- 2 tbsp. additional olive oil, and a little extra for brushing

- 2 cups risotto orecchiette (6 ounces)

- 2 tbsp. butter (unsalted)

- 1 minced shallot

- 2 minced garlic cloves

- 1/2 cup decreased sodium broth or chicken stock

- 4 cups baby arugula, sealed (4 ounces)

- 1 tbsp. lemon juice, freshly squeezed

- 1/2 cup Parmigiano-Reggiano cheese, grated

Instructions:

1. A big pot of water (salted) should be brought to a boil. Prepare a barbecue pan by preheating it. Double-skewer your scallops, shrimp, & cherry tomatoes with 8 sets of wooden skewers. Season with pepper and salt after brushing with olive oil.

2. Cook your pasta until it is al dente in the hot broth. Reserve 1/2 cup of the boiling water after draining the pasta.

3. Grill your kebabs over a high flame for about 7 minutes, rotating once, till browned and cooked through.

4. Meanwhile, melt your butter inside the two tbsp. of the olive oil in a big skillet. Cook, stirring

continuously until the shallot & garlic are softened, around 2 minutes over high heat. Boil for 3 minutes, or until your chicken broth has been reduced by half. Season with pepper and salt, pasta, lemon juice, cheese and arugula in the skillet. Toss with a few teaspoons of the allocated pasta water till your arugula is moderately wilted. Serve it, including seafood kebabs right away.

5. Spicy tequila butter on grilled oysters

Cook Time: 6 minutes

Serving: 6 people

Difficulty: Easy

Ingredients:

- Fennel seeds, 1/2 tsp.

- 1/4 tsp. red pepper smashed

- 7 tbsp. butter (unsalted)

- 1/4 cup tiny to medium spice leaves for garnish, including 36 tiny leaves

- 1 tsp. oregano, dried

- 2 tbsp. lemon juice, freshly squeezed

- Tequila (2 tbsp.)

- Kosher salt

- Serving salt (rock salt)

- 3 dozen scrubbed medium oysters

Instructions:

1. Toast your fennel seeds & smashed red pepper inside a skillet over medium heat for 1 minute or until fragrant. Allow cooling entirely before transferring to a mortar. Crush your ingredients to a smooth paste with a spatula and move to a dish.

2. Cook 3 1/2 tbsp. butter in the same skillet over medium heat for 2 minutes, or until it begins to brown. Cook, changing once, until the sage is crisp, about 2 minutes. Move your sage to a dish using a slotted spoon. In the same bowl as the spices, add the browned sugar. Continue with the leftover butter & 36 herb leaves, reserving the leaves to garnish.

3. Fill the mortar with the initial set of cooked sage leaves & break them with the ladle. Season it with salt after adding oregano, tequila and lemon juice to the butter. Keep it warm.

4. Preheat the grill. Using rock salt, cover a platter. Grill your oysters over medium temperature for 1 - 2 minutes or till they open. Remove the top shell from the oysters and drop them over the rock salt, becoming vigilant to not leak their liquor. Serve the oysters with a dollop of soft tequila butter and a crisp sage leaf on top.

6. Squid with citrus and soy

Cook Time: 15 minutes

Serving: 4 people

Difficulty: Easy

Ingredients:

- 1 tbsp. mirin

- 1 tbsp. soy sauce

- 1/3 cup new lemon juice or yuzu juice

- 2 cups of water

- 2-pound squid tentacles preserved, 1 inch of thick crosswise cut

Instructions:

1. Merge the soy sauce, water, yuzu juice and mirin into a mixing cup.

2. Refrigerate part of your marinade in an enclosed tub for future use. Attach the squid to the tub with the leftover marinade and set aside for more than 30 minutes or till 4 hours at room temp.

3. Preheat the barbecue. Squid can be drained. Grill for 3 minutes over medium-high heat, rotating once, till tender & white throughout. Serve immediately.

7. Miso-chile butter grilled lobsters

Cook Time: 28 minutes

Serving: 4 people

Difficulty: Easy

Ingredients:

- 1 cubed unsalted butter stick

- 2 tbsp. white miso

- 1 tbsp. Sriracha chili sauce

- 2 tbsp. lemon juice, with lemon wedges for consumption

- 2 scallions bunches

- 1 tbsp. rapeseed oil

- Pepper

- 1 tbsp. rapeseed oil

- Kosher salt

- 8 metal skewers, long

- 4 1/2 pound lobsters, divided lengthwise with claws removed and set aside

Instructions:

1. Melt your butter in a shallow saucepan. Combine the miso, sriracha, & lemon juice in a mixing bowl. 1/4 cup butter is set aside for serving.

2. Preheat the grill. Toss your scallions, including the oil in a big mixing bowl & season with pepper and salt. 5 minutes over the mild sun, rotating once, till lightly charred & tender. Toss 1 tbsp. of your miso-chile with the scallions.

3. To hold the bodies of lobster upright, skewer them from their tail to its head. 2 tbsp. of miso, chile butter, brushed over lobster meat Turn and bast the lobster claws and bodies with the residual miso chile butter with low heat till the shells are light red, for 7 - 8 mins for its tails & 12 - 15 mins for its claws. Strip the skewers from the skewers.

4. Scatter your scallions on top of your lobsters over the platter or bowls. Serve it with the lemon

wedges & the 1/4 cup of miso chile butter that was set aside.

8. Horseradish tabasco sauce on pop open clams

Cook Time: 5 minutes

Serving: 4 people

Difficulty: Easy

Ingredients:

- 4 tsp. softened unsalted butter

- 2 tsp. horseradish, drained

- 1 tsp. Tabasco sauce

- 1/4 tsp. lemon zest, finely grated

- 1 tbsp. lemon juice, freshly squeezed

- 1/4 tsp. pimentón a la Vera

- Salt

- 2 dozen scrubbed littleneck clams

- For serving, grilled pieces of crumbly white bread

Instructions:

1. Preheat the grill. Combine the butter, including the horseradish, lemon zest, pimentón de la Vera and tabasco in a shallow tub. Season it with salt.

2. Grill your clams on high heat for around 25 seconds or before they pop up. Carefully flip the clams around until the meat part is down, using tongs. Cook for another 20 seconds, or before the clam liquids begin to boil. Place the clams in a serving tub and set them aside. Serve it with grilled bread & about 1/2 tsp. of horseradish Tabasco sauce on top of every clam.

9. Grilled veggies al cartoccio and shellfish

Cook Time: 40 minutes

Serving: 4 people

Difficulty: Medium

Ingredients:

- Broccoli, 1 bunch

- 8 spears of fat asparagus

- 8 tiny carrots with a bit of stem

- 8 big red radishes, halved lengthwise with few stems attached

- 4 medium onions, crosswise halved

- 1 red onion, sliced from the root end into about 1/2-inch thick wedges

- The drizzle of additional olive oil

- Salt

- 16 tiny oysters scrubbed, like Wellfleet

- 16 scrubbed littleneck clams

- Scrubbed mussels (24 big mussels)

- 4 basil sprigs, big

- Serve with warm crusty bread

Instructions:

1. Preheat the grill. Mix each vegetable with the olive oil and salt in a big mixing cup. Remove the broccoli & grill until finely charred, around 1 minute each hand, over medium-high heat. Place on a wide tray. Remove the asparagus & carrots from the grill & grill for around 1 minute, or till mildly charred; switch to a dish. Cut the sides down, grill your radishes, onion wedges and tomatoes till mildly charred, around 2 minutes. Toss along with the rest of the vegetables.

2. Take 8 16x18-inch bits of high-duty aluminum foil and rip them apart. Pair the sheets and place them on top of each other. Drizzle the olive oil over the oysters, mussels and clams in four sets of foil. Drizzle additional olive oil over the vegetables and put them on top of the shellfish. Toss each

with a tbsp. of water, 1 basil sprig, and 1 pinch of salt. Fold that foil into tidy rectangular packages by wrapping it securely.

3. Place the packs on your grill and arrange them as needed. Cover & cook over medium-high heat, stirring once or twice, for around 25 minutes, or till the packages are puffed & sizzling. Serve directly with bread.

10. Apple-grilled shrimp with charred scallions

Cook Time: 5 minutes

Serving: 8 people

Difficulty: Easy

Ingredients:

- 2 1/2 teaspoons additional olive oil and 1/4 cup

- Sherry vinegar, 1 tbsp.

- 1 tbsp. lime juice, freshly squeezed

- 1/2 tsp. smoked paprika, sweet

- 1/2 tsp. mustard (Dijon)

- Season with salt & freshly ground pepper.

- Scallions, 6

- 1 pound regular shelled & deveined shrimp

- 1 cored, julienned and peeled Granny Smith apple

- 1 tbsp. sesame seeds, toasted

Instructions:

1. Whisk together 1/4 cup and one tbsp. of olive oil, lime juice, mustard, vinegar and paprika in a small bowl. Season with pepper and salt in the dressing.

2. Caramelize the scallions in a big saucepan having boiling salted water for 1 minute, or until bright orange. Drain your scallions and rinse them with cold water before patting them dry.

3. Preheat the grill. Season your scallions with pepper and salt after rubbing them with 1/2 tbsp. Olive oil. Season the shrimp with pepper and salt and toss with the leftover 1 tbsp. of the olive oil

in a tub. Grill your scallions for 30 seconds on each side over high temperature until finely charred. Grill your shrimp for around 1 minute on each side or until finely charred & white throughout.

4. Chuck the apple and 1 tbsp. of the seasoning in a moderate tub. Grilled scallions can be cut into around 2-inch of lengths. Organize your shrimp over the top of the scallions & apple over a platter. Serve with the leftover dressing drizzled over your shrimp & sesame seeds sprinkled on top.

11. Arugula & melon salad with grilled squid

Cook Time: 5 minutes

Serving: 6 people

Difficulty: Easy

Ingredients:

- 1 pound baby squid, washed

- 1/2 tsp. lemon zest, finely grated

- 1/2 tsp. lime zest, finely grated

- 1/2 tsp. orange zest, finely grated

- 1 1/4 tsp. red pepper smashed

- 1 cup of extra olive oil

- 2 cups parsley berries, flat-leaf (coarsely chopped)

- 6 fillets of anchovies

- 4 garlic cloves, big (smashed)

- 2 tsp. capers, drained

- 1 shallot, broad (chopped)

- Red wine vinegar, 2 tbsp.

- Freshly roasted black pepper and sea salt

- 2 tbsp. freshly squeezed lemon juice

- 4 oz. arugula kid

- 3 cups cubed cantaloupe (around 1 pound)

- 2 celery ribs from the inside (thinly sliced)

- 1 tiny red chile, young and spicy (thinly sliced)

Instructions:

1. Open these quid bodies on the surface you are working by splitting them lengthwise. Transfer it to the tub and mark a crosshatch design on the insides. Combine the tentacles, 1 tsp. red pepper flakes, 1/4 cups olive oil and citrus zest in a mixing dish. 1 hour in the refrigerator

2. Meanwhile, pulse the parsley, garlic, shallot, anchovies and capers inside a food processor till finely chopped. Pulse in 1/2 cup olive oil until a rough puree form. Season your salsa verde with pepper and salt, then include the vinegar & the leftover 1/4 tsp. crushed red pepper.

3. Preheat the grill or the grill pan. Salt and spice the squid. Grill for 5 minutes over high fire, rotating once, till charred in patches. Move the bodies of the squid to a cutting board and slice them thinly. Toss part of a salsa verde with the squid in a medium mixing dish.

4. Season it with salt and whisk the leftover 1/4 cup olive oil and lemon juice in a big mixing bowl. Toss gently with the arugula, celery, melon & fresh chile. Toss in the squid once more. Serve the leftover salsa verde with the salad on a platter or bowls.

12. Lemony soy shrimp & scallops

Cook Time: 5 minutes

Serving: 16 people

Difficulty: Easy

Ingredients:

- 1 1/2 cup soy sauce (low sodium)

- 1 tablespoon mirin

- 1-quart sake

- 2 lemons, cut very thinly

- 2 jalapenos, cut very thinly

- 1 pound regular shelled & deveined shrimp

- Big sea scallops, 1 pound

- Vegetable oil

Instructions:

1. Integrate your soy sauce, sake, jalapenos, mirin and lemon slices in the ceramic baking plate or a glass.

2. String your shrimp into eight bamboo skewers & place them in the marinade, rotating to evenly coat them. Go along the scallops in the same manner. Drain the seafood after 30 minutes in the refrigerator, turning when halfway in.

3. Grates should be oiled, and a barbecue should be lit. Rub the shrimp & scallops along with grill and oil until mildly charred, for about 4 minutes, rotating once or maybe twice. Serve instantly.

13. Feta-dill mixture with shrimp & lemon skewers

Cook Time: 5 minutes

Serving: 6 people

Difficulty: Easy

Ingredients:

- 1/2 cup low-fat plain yogurt

- 1 scallion, thinly cut white & light green pieces only

- 4 big garlic cloves, chopped very finely

- 2 1/2 tbsp. dill, finely chopped

- 1/2 cup feta cheese, crumbled (2 ounces)

- Season with salt & freshly ground pepper.

- 1 quarter cup of additional olive oil

- 2 lemons, sliced into twelve wedges each

- 2 pound big shrimp, peeled & deveined

Instructions:

1. Preheat the grill. Combine the yogurt, scallion, 1/4 tbsp. garlic, and 1/2 tbsp. dill in a regular mixing cup. Mix in your feta, slightly mashing it in. Salt & pepper to taste.

2. Merge the leftover minced garlic & 2 tbsp. of dill along with olive oil in a big mixing cup. Season

with pepper and salt & stir to coat the shrimp & lemons. On each of the 12 skewers, string 4 shrimp & 2 lemon wedges. Season with pepper and salt and fry, regularly rotating, over a moderate fire till the shrimps are crispy & cooked through around 5 minutes. Move your skewers to a platter & cover it with your feta sauce right away.

14. Honeydew avocado salsa with grilled scallops

Cook Time: 8 minutes

Serving: 4 people

Difficulty: Easy

Ingredients:

- 2 tbsp. lime juice, freshly diced lime zest

- 1 tbsp. extra-virgin olive oil, plus a little extra for drizzling

- 2 1/2 cups of honeydew melon, rind extracted and sliced into around 1/4-inch dice

- 1 avocado, chopped into around 1/4-inch cubes

- Salt and black pepper, freshly ground

- Big sea scallops weighing 2 pounds

Instructions:

1. Preheat the grill. Mix your lime zest & juice with 1 tbsp. olive oil in a large mixing cup. Place in the sliced honeydew melon & avocado with a rubber spoon. Season your salsa with black pepper and salt.

2. Season your scallops with black pepper and salt after drizzling them with olive oil. 3 till 4 minutes each side over medium-high heat, rotating once, till nicely charred & only cooked through. Move your scallops in plates and serve with the salsa on the side.

15. Grilled greek scallops sandwiches

Cook Time: 5 minutes

Serving: 4 people

Difficulty: Easy

Ingredients:

• Greek-style full-milk yogurt, 1/4 cup

• 1 pinch of crumbled saffron threads

• 1 1/2 tsp. rice vinegar

• Freshly roasted pepper and sea salt

• 1 thinly sliced tiny black plum

• Additional olive oil

• 12 big sea scallops (approximately 1 1/4 pound)

• 2 thin prosciutto slices, sliced into small strips

• 36 tendrils of pea (1 cup)

Instructions:

1. Preheat the grill. Combine the saffron, vinegar and yogurt in a mixing bowl & season it with pepper and salt.

2. Rub the slices of plum with grill and oil for around 30 seconds on each side over high temperature until finely charred. Rub your scallops with the oil, season with pepper and salt, & grill these in high heat for around 1.5 minutes on each side, or until crispy and only cooked through.

3. Each scallop should be cut in equal parts crosswise. On the lower half of every scallop, place a plum slice. Place your prosciutto strips on top of the plums, and top with two pea tendrils & the scallop tips. Place 3 toothpicks on every plate and secure with toothpicks.

4. 1 tsp. Of your yogurt, the sauce should be spread on every scallop sandwich, and the leftover pea tendrils should be garnished. Serve with a drizzle of olive oil and a pinch of salt.

16. Simple grilled paella

Cook Time: 30 minutes

Serving: 6 people

Difficulty: Easy

Ingredients:

• 3 cups of fish stock or minimum sodium broth of chicken

• Shelled & deveined 1/2 pound big shrimp, shells set aside

• A pinch of crumbled saffron threads

• Half a lemon

• 2 tbsp. additional olive oil

• 6 ounces chorizo (about 2 tiny links), cut into 1/2 inch thick

• 2 finely sliced ripe tomatoes

• 2 minced garlic cloves

• 1 tsp. paprika (smoked)

• 1 1/2 cups arborio or calasparra rice (around 10 ounces)

• 1/2 pound washed squid, sliced into around 2-inch parts after halving lengthwise and scoring in a crosshatch pattern.

• 1 pound scrubbed cockles

• Big lump crab, 1/2 pound

• 1 cup (5 ounces) red roasted peppers, sliced into strips

• 2 tbsp. parsley, chopped

• Serving with hot sauce & lemon wedges

Instructions:

1. Mix the stock, shrimp shells, & saffron in a big saucepan. Squeeze half of the lemon into the saucepan & heat to a boil. Enable to cool for about 10 minutes after withdrawing from the sun. Drop the solids from the broth & discard them.

2. In the meantime, preheat the barbecue. Preheat your olive oil inside a big flameproof skillet over the grill. Cover the pan & cover the grill after adding the chorizo. Cook for around 5 minutes over high temperature or till your chorizo is crackling & finely browned. Cover your skillet with the tomatoes, smoked paprika, and garlic and simmer, mixing once and even twice, till the tomatoes become softened around 5 minutes. Stir in the rice to coat it in the tomato sauce. Add your shrimp broth and blend well. Cover the pan, cover the grill, and simmer for 10 minutes or till most of your broth gets consumed. Combine the lobster, squid, and cockles in a mixing dish. Cover the pan, close the oven, & cook for around 8 minutes, or till the rice becomes al dente & a crust has grown on the underside of the skillet, & your seafood is fried. Cook, constantly stirring, until the crab, peppers, & parsley are thoroughly cooked. Serve with lemon wedges and spicy sauce.

17. Tacos with spiced crab

Cook Time: 25 minutes

Serving: 4 people

Difficulty: Easy

Ingredients:

- 2 finely diced medium tomatoes

- 2 big red radishes, diced to 1/4 inch

- 1 finely chopped tiny red onion

- 1/4 cup cilantro, chopped

- Sriracha chile sauce, 2 tsp.

- Salt

- 1 jalapeno, big

- 1 bell pepper in red color, diced into third-inch cubes

- 1 bell pepper in yellow color, diced into third-inch cubes

- 3 tbsp. additional olive oil

- 1 tbsp. lime juice, freshly squeezed

- 1 tbsp. mint leaves, chopped

- 1/2 pounds of lump crabmeat with shells removed

- Halved or quartered 810-inches flour tortillas

Instructions:

1. Combine the radishes, 2 tbsp. cilantro, sriracha, tomatoes and red onion in a regular mixing bowl. Include salt in your salsa.

2. Preheat the grill pan or light the grill. Over mild heat, turn the jalapeno until it is fully charred. Allow that to cool completely before discarding the skin of charred, stem, & seeds. Chop the jalapeno finely.

3. Combine the yellow and red bell peppers, lime juice, mint, the leftover 2 tbsp. of cilantro, jalapeno and olive oil in a medium mixing cup. Season it with salt and carefully roll in your crabmeat.

4. Grill your tortillas for around 20 seconds on each side over a high flame or till puffed & crispy in patches. Hot tortillas & salsa go along with the spiced crab.

18. Miso butter-grilled shrimp

Cook Time: 14 minutes

Serving: 4 people

Difficulty: Easy

Ingredients:

- 1 softened piece unsalted butter

- 2 tbsp. white miso

- 1 tbsp. new lemon juice, grated finely

- 1 tbsp. scallion, thinly cut, additional for garnish

- Big shelled & deveined shrimp, 1 pound

- 2 tbsp. oil (canola)

- 1 big minced garlic clove

- 1 tsp. gochugaru (a chile powder of Korea) and other such chile powder

- 1 tsp. salt (kosher)

- 1 1/2 tsp. brined marinated mustard seeds (from a pan of pickles)

Instructions:

1. Combine your butter, adding the miso, lemon juice and lemon zest in a food processor and puree till it gets smooth. Include the one tbsp. of scallion & pulse until it is completely incorporated. Put aside the miso butter in a big mixing bowl.

2. Mix your shrimp with garlic, salt, oil and chile powder in a separate big mixing bowl and set aside for around 10 minutes.

3. Preheat the grill pan or light the grill. Grill your shrimp at high temperature, rotating once, for around 4 minutes, or till almost cooked through. Toss the shrimp in your miso butter right away till it is well cooked. Serve the shrimp garnished with scallions, brine and mustard seeds (pickled).

Chapter 4: Grilled poultry recipe

1. Best grilled chicken breast

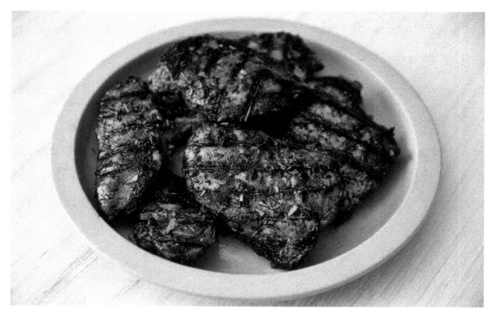

Cook Time: 15 minutes

Serving: 4 people

Difficulty: Easy

Ingredients:

- 1/4 cup of balsamic vinegar

- Additional olive oil, 3 tbsp.

- Brown sugar, 2 tbsp.

- 3 garlic cloves, minced

- 1 tsp. thyme (dried)

- 1 tsp. rosemary (dried)

- 4 breasts of chickens

- Kosher salt

- Black pepper, freshly ground

- Parsley, freshly chopped, to use as a garnish

Instructions:

1. Whisk together the balsamic vinegar, brown sugar, dried herbs, olive oil and garlic in a moderate mixing bowl, seasoning thoroughly with pepper and salt. 1/4 cup should be set aside.

2. Toss the chicken in the bowl to mix. Allow at least for 20 minutes & until overnight to marinate.

3. Preheat the grill to medium-high temperature. Add the chicken to the grill and cook for 6 minutes on each side, basting with the reserved marinade.

Before eating, garnish with parsley.

2. Grilled honey chicken

Cook Time: 30 minutes

Serving: 4 people

Difficulty: Easy

Ingredients:

- 2 tbsp. margarine or butter

- 1/3 cup of honey

- 1 tbsp. of lemon juice

- 1/3 cup of honey

- 4 chicken breast pieces, skinless and boneless

Instructions:

1. Preheat the grill to medium temperature.

2. In a pan over medium heat, melt the butter. Cook for around1 to 2 minutes until the garlic is fragrant. Honey & lemon juice must be whisked in. Half is set aside for basting, & the other part is brushed onto the breasts of the chicken.

3. Place your chicken over the grill after lightly oiling the grate. Cook it for around 6 - 8 minutes on each hand, flipping halfway through. In the last five minutes, baste often. When the placed meat becomes firm and the juices flow out, the chicken is cooked.

3. Grilled filipino chicken

Cook Time: 30 minutes

Serving: 8 people

Difficulty: Easy

Ingredients:

- 3 cups of water

- 1 cup of apple cider vinegar or coconut vinegar

- 1/2 cup freshly squeezed lemon juice

- 1/2 cup of soy sauce or tamari

- A quarter cup of fish sauce (asian)

- 10 crushed garlic cloves

- 2 tsp. of sugar

- 1 tbsp. red pepper, crushed

- 1 tsp. black peppercorns

- 5 full star anise pods

- 5 leaves of bay

- 2 chickens of 3 1/2 pounds, each sliced into 8 bits

- Brushing with canola oil

- Kosher salt

- Black pepper, freshly roasted

Instructions:

1. Combine every ingredient, except for the salt, pepper and oil, in a big, durable resalable plastic container. Seal your bag, pushing out all the air, and shake to equally spread the chicken & adobo marinade. Refrigerate for at least one hour.

2. Remove your chicken from the marinade and set it aside. Allow the chicken & make it stand for around 30 minutes at room temperature after patting it dry.

3. In the meantime, preheat the grill. Season your chicken with black pepper and salt after brushing it with oil. Grill over mild heat, frequently rotating, for around 30 minutes, or until mildly charred & an immediate read thermometer placed in the thickest bits registers 165°. Until serving, move your chicken on a plate and set aside for 10 minutes to rest.

4. Basil chicken & zucchini on the grill

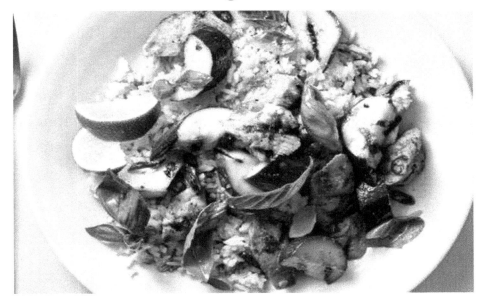

Cook time: 6 minutes

Serving: 4 people

Difficulty: Easy

Ingredients:

- 1 cup rice, white

- 1 lime, including serving wedges

- 2 garlic cloves

- 1 tbsp. soy sauce (low sodium)

- 1/2 tsp. of sugar

- 1/2 thinly cut red chile

- 4 tiny zucchini, halved lengthwise (approximately 1 1/4 pound)

- 2 tbsp. extra virgin olive oil, split

- Kosher salt & pepper

- 1 lb. of chicken tenders

- 2 and a half cup of basil, finely chopped

Instructions

1. Cook the rice according to the box instructions.

2. Squeeze 2 tbsp. of lime juice into a big mixing bowl after zesting the lime. In a mixing cup, finely grind the garlic, and then add the soy sauce, chile and sugar.

3. 1 tbsp. of oil, 1/4 tsp. of salt, and 1/4 tsp. of pepper, brushed on zucchini. Season chicken tenders with 1/4 tsp. of salt & pepper and the leftover tbsp. of oil. Switch to the cutting board after grilling zucchini till just slightly tender & chicken till it is almost cooked through, around 3 minutes each side.

4. Toss the zucchini & chicken in the sauce, then add in the basil & serve rice with the lime wedges.

5. Coconut Lime Slaw with Grilled Chicken

Cook time: 5 minutes

Serving: 4 people

Difficulty: Easy

Ingredients:

- 8 chicken cutlets, small

- Kosher salt & pepper

- A single lime

- Coconut oil, 3 tbsp.

- 1 tsp. of sugar

- 1/2 tsp. of fish sauce

- 1 lb. of thinly sliced red cabbage

- 2 scallions, matchstick-sized

- 1 tbsp. of cilantro

Instructions:

1. Preheat the grill to moderate temperatures.

2. Sprinkle salt and black pepper on the chicken. Grill for 3 minutes, rotating once, till just cooked completely.

3. In the meantime, zest the lime and set it aside in a small tub. 1 tbsp. of lime juice, squeezed into a big mixing bowl. Combine the coconut milk, fish sauce in a mixing bowl. Stir in the sugar until it dissolves, then mix in the cabbage & scallions until they are finely covered.

4. Sprinkle lime zest on the chicken as it comes off the grill. Serve the chicken & slaw on separate bowls. Serve the slaw with a garnish of cilantro.

6. Grilled Sesame-Ginger Chicken Breasts

Cook Time: 12 minutes

Serving: 4 people

Difficulty: Easy

Ingredients:

- 4 boneless chicken breasts (around 4 - 6 ounces per)

- Marinade Ingredients:

- A half-cup of soy sauce

- 3 cloves of garlic (peeled & crushed)

- 1/4 cup of rice wine vinegar, flavored

- Honey (2 tbsp.)

- 1 tbsp. ginger root (fresh) (peeled and grated)

- 4 green onions, medium (chopped)

- 2 tsp. sesame seed, toasted

- 1 tsp. sesame seeds, toasted

- 2 tsp. whole cilantro leaves as a garnish

Instructions:

1. To make your marinade, add the garlic, ginger, sesame oil, sesame seeds, soya sauce, vinegar, onions and honey in a large plastic zipper container.

2. Seal the bag securely after adding the breasts of the chicken and pressing out any excess air. Refrigerate the bag for around 30 - 60 minutes, and then take it out of the refrigerator for about 20 minutes prior you intend to plan cooking.

3. Prepare the grill pan or a grill. Spray with the cooking spray of canola and turn the flame up to maximum.

4. Remove the chicken placed in the marinade and set it aside. 6 minutes each side on the grill, till tender and thoroughly cooked. Serve it with the cilantro leaves as a garnish.

7. Jerk Chicken, (Jamaican)

Cook Time: 20 minutes

Serving: 5 people

Difficulty: Easy

Ingredients:

• Skinless breasts of chicken, 900 grams/ 2 pounds

• 1 pepper, jalapeno (seeded & diced)

• 45 ml water (3 tbsp.)

• 1 lime juice

• 1 big lemon juice

• 1 tbsp. dijon mustard (15 mL)

• 2 garlic cloves (minced)

• 2 bouillon cubes (chicken)

• 1 tsp. dried parsley (5 mL)

• 1 tsp. (5 mL) cumin powder

• 2.5 ml dried thyme, 1/2 teaspoon

• 1/2 tsp. of cinnamon or allspice (2.5 mL)

- 1/2 tsp. of black pepper (2.5 mL)

- A dash of the cinnamon

Instructions:

1. In a small resalable plastic container or baking dish, combine all the ingredients except for the chicken. Toss in the chicken and toss to cover.

2. Cover and refrigerate for around 30 minutes - 1 hour so that it can be marinated in jerk seasoning. Preheat the grill to high. Remove the chicken from the jerk marinade & place it in the saucepan.

3. Boil it. Put the chicken on the grill and cook for about 7 - 10 minutes on each side (or till it is done), basting with the leftover jerk marinade.

8. Grilled crispy chicken

Cook Time: 6 minutes

Serving: 4 people

Difficulty: Easy

Ingredients:

- 1 tsp. dried thyme leaves

- 1 tsp. of chives (dried)

- Basil leaves, 1/2 tsp. (dried)

- Bread crumbs (1/2 cup) (dry, fine, purchased)

- 1/4 cup of grated Parmesan

- A half tsp. of salt

- 1/8 tsp. of pepper

- 1 tsp. of extra virgin olive oil

- 4 chicken breasts, boneless and skinless

- A single egg (beaten)

Instructions:

1. Prepare a grill with two sides. Combine the bread crumbs, salt, pepper, herbs and grated cheese in a deep pan. Drizzle your olive oil on the crumbs and slowly push it in till they are evenly covered.

2. Place the chicken breasts around 2 waxed paper sheets. Slightly pound the chicken breasts with the rolling pin or meat mallet till they get 1/2 inch thick.

3. On a table, there are chicken breasts.

4. Chicken breasts should be dipped in a beating egg.

5. Then press every coated breast further into the mixture of breadcrumb.

6. Cook the breast of the chicken for almost 4 - 6 minutes on a 2-sided double indoor grill or until fully cooked to around 160 F & juices run clear.

9 Easy grilled chicken with rosemary and lemon

Cook Time: 40 minutes

Serving: 4 people

Difficulty: Medium

Ingredients:

- 2 divided broiler chickens (approximately 5 - 6 pounds total)

- 1/4 cup of vegetable oil

- Melted butter (1/2 cup)

- Lemon juice, 1/3 cup

- 2 tsp. crushed dry rosemary

- 1 garlic clove, tiny

- 1 tsp. black pepper, freshly roasted, to taste

Instructions:

1. Collect the required ingredients.

2. Place the oiled rack 4 - 6 inches over medium coals to prepare your grill.

3. Combine the olive oil, lemon juice, garlic, salt, butter and rosemary in a large mixing bowl. 1/4

cup seasoned fat, brushed inside & out on the chicken

4. Place your chickens over the grill having the bone part down.

5. Turn the chicken halves every ten mins and baste them with the leftover butter mixture.

6. Grill for a total of about 30 - 40 minutes, or till the chicken gets tender & juices run purely until a fork pierced.

10. Bruschetta Chicken

Cook Time: 20 minutes

Serving: 4 people

Difficulty: Easy

Ingredients:

Bruschetta Topping:

- 6 seeded & diced plum tomatoes

- 1 cup fresh pearl-sized mozzarella balls

- 2 garlic cloves, minced

- 2 tbsp. olive oil (extra virgin)

- 1/4 cup of fresh basil, torn

- 1/4 tsp. of salt

- 1/4 tsp. black pepper, freshly ground

- Chicken breasts with Seasonings:

- 2 tsp. of seasoning (Italian)

- 1 tsp. of powdered garlic

- A half tsp. of salt

- 1/4 tsp. of black pepper, freshly ground

- 4 chicken breast pieces, boneless and skinless

- 2 tsp. of extra virgin olive oil

- Balsamic glaze to vincotto to serve

Instructions:

1. Collect the required ingredients.

2. Toss the sliced plum tomatoes, diced garlic, 2 tbsp. of fresh basil, olive oil, salt & new ground pepper in a regular mixing cup. Combine all ingredients in a mixing bowl and cool before ready to eat.

3. Combine the garlic powder, black pepper and salt in a tiny bowl. Using paper towels, pat your chicken breasts dry.

4. Brush 1 tbsp. of olive oil on each side of your chicken breasts & season each side with a prepared seasoning mix.

5. In a big skillet, melt leftover 1 tbsp. of olive oil over moderately high heat. Cook for around 6 to 8 minutes on each side, or till the chicken is cooked through and no more pink in color.

Chicken Bruschetta:

1. Allow your chicken to settle for around 5 minutes on a board of cutting before plating.

2. Place the ready-made bruschetta topping on top of your chicken breasts.

3. Serve with a balsamic glaze or vincotto drizzled on top.

4. With hot toasted crostini & a bottle of the favorite Italian wine, this dish is perfect.

11. Tasty bbq grilled chicken thighs

Cook Time: 50 minutes

Serving: 6 people

Difficulty: Medium

Ingredients:

• 4 pound of bone-in and skin-on chicken thighs

To marinade:

• 3 tbsp. of white vinegar

• 1 tbsp. salt (kosher)

• 1 tbsp. sugar (granulated)

• 1 tsp. crushed fake pepper

To make the barbecue sauce:

- Ketchup, 1 cup

- 1 tbsp. white vinegar

- 1/4 cup of brown sugar, packed

- 2 tbsp. of paprika (sweet)

- 1 tbsp. extra virgin olive oil

- 1 tbsp. chili powder

- 1 tsp. garlic powder

- Optional: 1 tsp. of cayenne pepper

- Kosher salt (1/2 tsp.)

Instructions:

1. To make the marinade, follow these steps:

2. Collect the required ingredients.

3. Using a paper towel, pat your chicken thighs off.

4. Mix together white vinegar, granulated sugar, red pepper, olive oil and salt in a big mixing bowl.

5. In the resalable plastic container, place the chicken thighs.

6. Pour the marinade over the top, close the container, and change to cover everything. Refrigerate for at least four hours and up to six hours.

7. Assemble the ingredients for your barbecue sauce:

8. In a shallow saucepan, mix together white vinegar, sweet paprika, chili powder, cayenne pepper, salt, brown sugar, olive oil and garlic powder.

9. Boil it, and then lower to low heat. Continue to cook for another 15 minutes on low heat, stirring regularly.

10. Remove the sauce from the heat & allow it to thicken for around 10 minutes before covering and setting it aside. Cool thoroughly before storing in an airtight jar in your refrigerator if preparing the sauce ahead of time. Before completing the recipe, make sure to get your sauce at room temperature, but do not overheat or boil it.

Grill your chicken:

1. Preheat a grill to around 300 F on a medium-low flame.

2 Remove the chicken from the marinade, discard the remaining marinade, & grill the thighs of your chicken skin-side down.

3. Cook for around 30 minutes, stirring periodically, with the cover down.

4. Brush the sauce over your chicken for the last twenty minutes or more of preparation or till the meat hits a core temperature of about 165 F & the sauce has thickened to a thick consistency. Be sure to check the accuracy of many pieces.

5. Remove your chicken, place it over the heat & put it on a big platter until it has finished cooking. Allow for a 10-minute rest period after covering with aluminum foil.

6. Serve with a side dish of your choice.

BBQ baked chicken variation:

1. Not every other person has a grill or loves to grill.

2. If you don't wish to be outdoors in the cold, you should make it in the winters. This is where this fried; grilled chicken comes in.

3. Preheat your oven to 400 F. Cover a 13 by 9-inch baking pans lightly with the cooking spray.

4. Remove the thighs from the marinade and put them down inside the tub, discarding the remaining marinade.

5. Bake it for 20 minutes. Reduce the heat to about 375 F.

6. Rub barbecue sauce on the thighs after carefully pouring off any excess fat & drippings. Flip the thighs over with tongs and spray the surfaces with the barbecue sauce.

7. Cook for the next 15 mins, basting every 5 min with the barbecue sauce. The thighs get finished as an immediate thermometer reads 165 F.

8. Serve with a side dish of your choice.

12. Chicken Salad in a Mediterranean Style

Cook Time: 10 times

Serving: 4 people

Difficulty: Easy

Ingredients:

To marinade:

- 1/2 cup of extra virgin olive oil

- 1/4 cup of lemon juice

- 1 tbsp. oregano, dried

- A half tsp. of salt

- 1/4 tsp. black pepper, medium

Salad Ingredients:

- 4 chicken breasts, skinless and boneless

- 2 cups salad greens (baby spinach or other)

- 1/2 onion, red (peeled & thinly sliced)

- 2 tbsp. halved cherry tomatoes

- A half-cup of black olives (halved and pitted)

- Feta cheese, 1/2 cup (crumbled)

- 4 rounds of pita bread

Ingredients:

1. Collect the required ingredients.

2. Mix together half a cup of olive oil, 1/4 cup of lemon juice, black pepper, salt and dried oregano in a big mixing bowl.

3. Half of the mixture should be held in a different tub for the coating. Add the leftover half of your marinade to the breasts of the chicken and cover them fully. Refrigerate for almost 1 hour, but not more than four hours, covered with plastic wrap.

4. Preheat the outdoor grill and/or an indoor grill tray to 400 F.

5. Cook for 5 minutes on one side, then flip & cook for another 5 minutes, just till the chicken is cooked thru & no more pink.

6. Slice your chicken in half lengthwise.

7. Toss the tiny spinach and perhaps other different salad greens, diced red onion, feta cheese, cherry tomatoes and olives in a different dish. Toss all along with the dressing.

8. Place your salad on the platter & cover with grilled chicken slices & toasted the pita bread.

13. Marsala Grilled Chicken

Cook Time: 15 minutes

Serving: 4 people

Difficulty: Easy

Ingredients:

- 4 breasts of chicken (boneless & skinless)

To make the Marsala Sauce:

- 80 ml/ 1/3 cup
- Marsala wine, 1/4 cup i.e. (60 mL)
- 60 mL/ 1/4 cup cold chicken stock
- 2 cans of mushrooms, 4 oz. /120 mL (drained)
- 1 prosciutto slice (diced)
- 30 mL/2 tsp. heavy cream
- 2 tsp. shallots/10 mL (minced)
- 4 garlic cloves (minced)
- 2 tsp. cornstarch (10 mL)
- A quarter teaspoon (1.25 mL) of black pepper
- 1 tsp. fresh parsley (5 mL) (minced)

For the chicken rub:

- Salt (1/2 teaspoon)

- 1/2 tsp. of dried oregano

- 1/2 tsp. of fried thyme

- 1/2 tsp. of dried parsley

- 1/4 tsp. of marjoram

- 1/4 garlic powder (1.25 mL)

- 1 tsp. (5 mL) black pepper, powdered

Instructions:

1. Brush the breasts of the chicken with olive oil.

2. Clean the chicken breasts with the rub combination.

3. Refrigerate it for around 20 - 30 minutes after covering.

4. Make your sauce while the chicken is in the marinating process. Melt butter in a regular saucepan overheat.

5. Increase the heat to high and add the prosciutto, cooking for 2 minutes.

6. Sauté the shallots & garlic until they are finely browned.

7. Combine the marsala wine, black pepper and mushrooms in a mixing bowl. Cook for 5 minutes at a low temperature.

8. Pour the chicken stock into a saucepan and dissolve the cornstarch in it. Stir until it is well blended.

9. Continue to cook till the mixture thickens, adding parsley & cream if required.

10. Remove from the heat and cover to keep warm.

11. Preheat the grill to medium-high. Oil your grill grates with the tongs, rolled paper towels, & a decent quality smoke level oil until the grill is up to the temperature & right before setting the chicken on it. Create two to three loops over the grates.

12. Grill the breasts of chicken for around 6 - 8 minutes on each side of the grill.

13. Turn every breast 90 degrees on your grill after around 3 - 4 minutes to make crisscross lines.

Remove the chicken from the grill when it has reached a core temperature of around 165 degrees F in its thickest region of the chicken breast.

14. 1/4 of your warmed marsala solution should be spooned over every breast before serving.

14. Chicken kabobs in greek style

Cook Time: 10 minutes

Serving: 4 people

Difficulty: Easy

Ingredients:

For your chicken:

- 1 pound breast of chicken (boneless and skinless, sliced into around 1-inch chunks)

- 2 garlic cloves (peeled & minced)

- 2 tbsp. freshly squeezed lemon juice

- 3 tsp. extra virgin olive oil

- 1 tsp. oregano, dried

- 1 tsp. kosher salt

- 1/2 tsp. black pepper, medium

- 1 red color bell pepper, chopped (sliced into around 1-inch chunks)

- 1 red onion, tiny (peeled & sliced into around 1-inch chunks)

To make the sauce:

- 1 cup simple Greek-style yogurt, full fat

- 1 garlic clove (peeled & finely grated or minced)

- 1 tbsp. extra virgin olive oil

- 1 tbsp. lemon juice, finely squeezed

- 1 English cucumber (seedless) (grated)

- 1 tbsp. chill (fresh) (chopped)

- Salt (for taste)

• Pepper (for taste)

Instructions:

Marinade for the Chicken

1. Collect the required ingredients.

2. Make the marinade for the chicken. In a big mixing bowl, combine the olive oil, black pepper, dried oregano and salt.

3. Toss in the chicken bits to dip them in the marinade. Refrigerate it for around 30 mins or 3 hours, covered.

Preparing the Chicken

1. Collect the required ingredients.

2. The chicken can be grilled on an outside grill, in an inside grill tub, or under your broiler in the oven. Preheat which method you're going to use.

3. Remove your chicken placed to marinade and alternate threading the bits onto 4 skewers with the chunks of bell pepper and red onion. If you're using the wooden skewers, then soak them inside water for some minutes prior to using them to avoid them on fire.

4. Place your chicken over the grill & cook for around 5 minutes, then flip and cook for another 5 minutes, or till the chicken is completely cooked through. Cook for around 10 mins or till the chicken is completely cooked through if broiling.

Bakeware made of glass Caution.

1. When broiling and adding liquid to the hot plate, avoid using glass bakeware because it could burst. Tempered glass components can & do crack, even though they are labeled as stove or heat resistant.

2. To make your tzatziki sauce, combine all of the ingredients in a mixing bowl.

3. Collect the required ingredients.

4. In a mixing dish, combine the greek style garlic, lemon juice and olive oil in a bowl.

Using the box grater, grate your cucumber and suck out the extra liquid.

5. Season with pepper and salt to taste after adding the diced cucumber and fresh dill to your yogurt mixture.

6. Serve your chicken skewers, adding the yogurt sauce, warm flatbread, and additional lemon halves on the side for those who want a little more citrus. Any excess tzatziki sauce should be kept refrigerated. Have fun.

15. Bulgogi Chicken

Cook Time: 5 minutes

Serving: 6 people

Difficulty: Easy

Ingredients:

- 2-pound chicken thighs, boneless and skinless

- 1/2 onion, red (finely chopped)

- 2 garlic cloves (finely chopped or grated)

- 1 slice (15 gram) fresh ginger

- 1/4 cup of scallion (finely chopped, whites only)

- 3 tbsp. of soy sauce

- 1 tbsp. gochujang

- 1 tbsp. of honey

- 1 tbsp. sesame oil, toasted

- 1/4 cup of mirin

- 1/4 cup of sesame seeds

- Green onion tops as a garnish (sliced)

Ingredients:

1. Collect the requisite ingredients.

2. Slice your chicken thighs around 1 - 2 inches wide & a few inches long segments. Simply break the legs equal lengthwise for narrower thighs.

3. In a big mixing cup, combine the remaining ingredients and stir well.

4. Stir your chicken strips into the marinade to cover them thoroughly. Refrigerate it for few hours

or overnight, covered.

5. For searing, prepare a grill.

6. Based on the thickness, grill your marinated chicken slices for 2 to 3 minutes on each side.

7. Shift to a platter until completely cooked & top it with the diced tops of green onion.

8. Serve instantly with some desired side dishes.

16. Grilled chicken quesadilla

Cook Time: 10 minutes

Serving: 4 people

Difficulty: Easy

Ingredients:

- 8 oz. chicken tenders

- 1/4 cup of water

- 2 teaspoons cilantro, chopped (chopped)

- 1 jalapeno sliced chili

- 1 tbsp. lime juice, freshly squeezed

- 1 tbsp. extra virgin olive oil

- 4 red onions slices (1/4 inches thick)

- 4 eggplant slices (1/4 inch thick slices)

- 8 flour tortillas with a diameter of 6 inches

- Monterey Jack cheese, 1/2 cup (grated)

- 1/2 cup cheddar cheese, grated (grated)

- 2 teaspoons oil (vegetable)

- Yogurt and sour cream (to serve)

Instructions:

1. In a shallow baking pan, position the chicken tenders.

2. In a mixer, mix 1/4 cup of water, sliced jalapeno, olive oil, cilantro and lime juice. Blend until creamy, and then season with salt & pepper to taste.

3. Cover your chicken tenders full in the marinade. Refrigerate for 4 hours after covering.

4. Preheat your grill to high.

5. Remove the chicken from the marinade * grill for 6 minutes or until completely cooked.

6. Brush your onion & eggplant with the oil and season with salt & pepper before grilling for 4 minutes, rotating once.

7. Cover tortillas in the foil put them on the grill's top rack as you prepare the rest of the ingredients.

8. In a mixing tub, combine the cheeses.

9. Remove all of the items from the barbecue.

10. Half of the tortillas should have around 1/4 cup cheese on them.

11. Top with the chicken, one onion slice, & one eggplant slice.

12. As if you were having a taco, cover with another tortilla.

13. Place tortillas on the grill & cook in low heat till cheese gets melted & golden brown.

17. Parmesan grilled chicken

Cook Time: 10 minutes

Serving: 4 people

Difficulty: Easy

Ingredients:

- 4 skinless & boneless chicken breasts

- 3 finely sliced Roma tomatoes

- 4 oz. /115 grams mozzarella cheese, thinly sliced

- Parmesan cheese, 1/4 cup (60 mL)

- Basil leaves, around 5 - 6

- 2 tsp. olive oil (10 mL)

- 1/2 tsp. salt (2.5 mL)

- Black pepper, 1/2 tsp. (2.5 mL)

Instructions:

1. Collect the requisite ingredients.

2. Preheat the grill to medium-high.

3. Pounded the chicken breasts to a thickness of around 1/4 inch.

4. Using olive oil, black pepper and salt, coat the chicken.

5. Cook the chicken for around 5 minutes on the grill.

6. Place cheese & slices of tomato on top of the chicken.

7. Cook for a total of 5 or 6 minutes more.

8. Remove the chicken from the heat when the inner temperature exceeds 165 F, set aside for around 1 - 2 minutes, then garnish with basil leaves before serving.

9. Make a chicken sandwich or eat it over pasta.

10. Have fun.

18. Cinnamon chicken on the grill

Cook Time: 20 minutes

Serving: 4 people

Difficulty: Easy

Ingredients:

- 1 chicken in a fryer (sliced into pieces)

- Dry sherry, 1/2 cup or 120 mL

- 80 ml honey, 1/3 cup

- 2 tsps. cinnamon powder

- 1 tsp. curry powder (5 mL)

Instructions:

1. In a mixing cup, combine the dry sherry, garlic salt, honey, curry powder and cinnamon.

2. Place the chicken inside the shallow baking pan and marinate it evenly.

3. Refrigerate for a minimum 1 hour before serving.

4. Preheat the grill.

5. Remove the chicken from the marinade and put it on the grill in medium heat for around 10 - 12 mins per hand.

6. Since your marinade for the following recipe contains honey, you'll want to look at your chicken when it's grilling to ensure it does not burn.

7. When the chicken hits a core temperature of around 165 F, remove it from the oven. Serve with a variety of side dishes.

19. Chicken tikka, grilled

Cook Time: 15 minutes

Serving: 8 people

Difficulty: Easy

Ingredients:

• 1 cup finely chopped new coriander leaves (cilantro), plus more to garnish

• 2 tsp. ginger paste

• Garlic paste (3 tbsp.)

• Garam masala, 3–4 tbsp.

• 6 peppercorns

• 1 tsp. of kosher salt, additional salt to taste

• 1/2 tsp. of food coloring in orange color (optional)

• 1 cup yogurt (plain)

• 1 kg/2 1/4 pound chicken breast (boneless, skinless sliced into around 2-inch)

• 1 onion, big (cut into rings)

• Lime juice (3 tbsp.) (freshly squeezed, lemon juice)

• 1 tsp. chaat masala, additional for taste

- For serving, use basmati rice.

- Wedges of lemon or lime as a garnish

Instructions:

1. Collect the requisite ingredients.

Chicken tikka, grilled

2. In the tub of the food processor, combine the ginger, garam masala, food coloring, garlic, salt and peppercorns. Scrap down the sides of the bowl as needed to create a smooth paste.

3. In the food processor, combine the spices.

4. With the silicone spatula, scrape your mixture in the large mixing cup, apply the yogurt, & season to taste. Toss in the chicken parts to coat. Refrigerate the bowl overnight, covered.

Tikka marinade

5. Thread your chicken onto the skewers, leaving room between each portion to ensure even cooking. Preheat the grill to a medium-high temperature or a rack on the top of an oven to 400 degrees F.

Skewers of chicken tikka

6. Put your skewers on your grill or in the oven having a tray under it to collect the drippings. Cook for 12 - 15 minutes, or till your chicken gets browned on both sides & tender.

Chicken tikka, grilled

7. Place the skewers on a plate to serve.

8. Take the chicken from the skewers and arrange it on a tray.

9. Place your onion rings inside a bowl & drizzle with lime juice. Mix in the chaat masala until your onions get fully covered. Serve the chicken with basmati rice or naan, topped with onions and the leftover coriander.

Chapter 5: Grilled Appetizers

1. Thai chicken satay

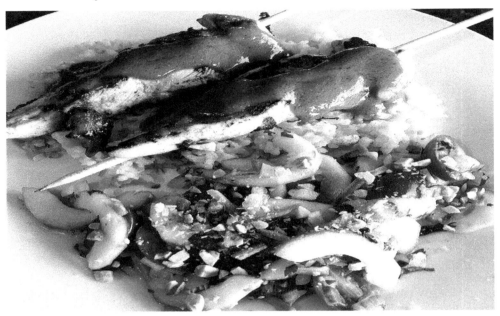

Cook time: 10 minutes

Serving: 4 people

Difficulty: Easy

Ingredients:

- 1/2 cup of coconut milk from a can

- 1/2 tsp. coriander powder

- 1 tsp. curry powder (yellow)

- 1 tsp. fish sauce

- 1/2 tbsp. chili oil

- 1 pound chicken breast pieces, skinless and boneless - sliced into strips

- 1 tbsp. new cilantro, chopped

- 1 tbsp. unsalted peanuts, diced

- 12 wooden drumsticks, soaked for around 15 minutes in water

- 1 cup thai peanut sauce (prepared)

Instructions:

1. Combine the ground coriander, fish sauce, chili oil, coconut milk and curry powder in a regular mixing dish. Stir in your chicken breast pieces to cover them. Refrigerate it for around 30 minutes and up to 2 hours, covered.

2. Preheat a grill, either indoors or outdoors, to high heat. Using skewers, thread your chicken strips. Remove the marinade and discard it.

3. 2 or 3 minutes a side on the barbecue, or before no more pink. The length of time can be determined by the thickness of your strips. Serve on a serving plate with peanuts and cilantro on top. Serve with a dipping sauce made from peanuts.

2. Grilled portobellos with pesto

Cook time: 20 minutes

Serving: 3 people

Difficulty: Easy

Instructions:

- 6 mushrooms, portobell

- 1 tbsp. extra virgin olive oil

- 1 minced tiny shallot

- 1 garlic clove, minced

- 1 tbsp. Chardonnay champagne, or to taste

- Pesto (3 tbsp.)

- Pine nuts, 2 tbsp.

12 cup shredded 3-cheese mix (Italian)

Instructions:

1. Remove the stems from the mushrooms and cut them finely.

2. Cook & stir the chopped mushroom heads, shallot, & garlic in the olive oil over medium temperature in the skillet until softened, around 5 minutes. Pour your wine in the skillet and roast, stirring constantly with the wooden spoon, till the liquid has evaporated, about 1 - 2 minutes.

Allow 10 minutes for the mixture to cool to room temperature.

3. Preheat the outdoor grill to medium heat & brush the grate gently with grease.

4. Brush your olive oil solution over the tops of each mushroom & put on the grilling pan, top side up. In a tub, combine the pesto, pine nuts, and mushroom stem mixed; feed into every mushroom. Over your filling, sprinkle the Italian cheese mix.

5. Grill the mushrooms on a preheated grill for around 10 minutes, or till the sides are blackened & the stuffing starts bubbling.

3. Delicious Garlic Grilled Bread

Cook time: 5 minutes

Serving: 10 people

Difficulty: Easy

Ingredients:

- 1 cup extra virgin olive oil

- 1 cup basil leaves, chopped

- 3 tsp. garlic, minced

- 1 loaf of calabrese bread (crumbly Italian bread) (8 ounces), sliced into around 1/2-inch slices

- Salt & coarsely black pepper

Instructions:

1. In a tub, combine the oil, basil, & garlic.

2. Preheat a medium-hot outdoor grill. Cook the slices of bread on your grill for 2 - 3 minutes, or till the underside is toasted. Using only 1/2 of your oil mixture, baste each grilled sides of the bread. Season with salt & pepper. 1 - 2 minutes on the grill before the bottoms get toasted.

3. Turn the bread slices over and baste with the leftover oil mixture.

4. Remove from the heat and season it with salt & pepper.

4. Eggplant rollups (grilled)

Cook time: 6 minutes

Serving: 4 people

Difficulty: Easy

Ingredients:

- 1 peeled eggplant, cut lengthwise into around 1/4-inch slices

- Salt to taste

- 1 tablespoon extra-virgin olive oil, or to taste

- 1 pinch of Italian seasoning

- 2 canned of whole charred red peppers, drained & diced

- 1 (four ounce) of log softened goat cheese

Instructions:

1. Sprinkle all sides of the eggplant slices with salt on a big pan. Refrigerate for around 30 minutes, or till all of the water was already taken out. Clean the eggplant slices by rinsing them and patting them dry with the help of paper towel.

2. Preheat the grill to medium heat & brush the grate gently with grease.

3. Season all sides of the eggplant slices with the Italian seasoning & a light coating of the olive oil.

4. Grill the eggplant slices for around 3 minutes each side on a preheated grill. On one side of every eggplant piece, spread the goat cheese and red pepper roasted. Serve the sandwiches open-faced or folded up.

5. Peach flatbread pizza with grilled prosciutto

Cook time: 29 minutes

Serving: 4

Difficulty: Easy

Ingredients:

- 1/4 cup honey

- 1 cup of balsamic vinegar

- 12 tbsp. lemon juice

- A quarter tsp. of black pepper

- 2 read of naan

- Ricotta cheese, 4 oz.

- 2 sliced new peaches

- 1 box (3 ounces) prosciutto, cut into bits

- 3 tsp. new basil, thinly sliced

Instructions:

1. In a shallow saucepan, combine honey, pepper, balsamic vinegar and lemon juice. Bring it to boil on high heat, and then reduce it to a low heat environment. Cook for around 15 minutes, or until the mixture get reduced to around 1/3 cup.

2. Gently grease the grill grate and preheat the outdoor grill to medium-high temperature.

3. Grill naan for 2 - 3 minutes, or until slight char marks surface. Ricotta cheese should be spread over the burnt edge. Peaches & prosciutto are served on top. Garnish with basil leaves. Drizzle the balsamic reduction over the top.

4. Put the flatbreads back on the grill. Grill, covered, for 7 minutes or till the cheese get melted & the base of your flatbread starts to burn.

6. Tofu skewers including sriracha sauce on the grill

Cook time: 10 minutes

Serving: 2 people

Difficulty: Easy

Ingredients:

- 1 zucchini, peeled and sliced into big chunks

- 1 big bell pepper in red color, peeled and cut into chunks

- 10 large of mushrooms

- 2 tbsp. garlic sauce srira

- 1/4 cup of soy sauce

- 2 tbsp. sesame seed oil

- 1/4 cup onion, diced

- 1 sliced jalapeno pepper

- Black pepper for taste

Instructions:

1. In a mixing tub, combine the tofu, red pepper, mushrooms and zucchini. In a shallow bowl, combine the soy sauce, onion, pepper, sriracha sauce, sesame oil and jalapeno; sprinkle over tofu & vegetables. Lightly toss to coat. Enable to marinate in your refrigerator for at around 1 hour.

2. Gently grease the grill grate and preheat the outdoor grill to medium-high temperature.

3. Skewer the tofu & vegetables together. Grill every skewer for 10 minutes, or until finished to your taste. Every leftover marinade can be used as the dipping sauce.

7. Bruschetta with strawberry goat cheese

Cook time: 15 minutes

Serving: 6 people

Difficulty: Easy

Ingredients:

- 1/2 cup of balsamic vinaigrette

- 12 Italian bread slices

- 1 tbsp. extra virgin olive oil

- 1 pound washed & diced strawberries

- 2 tbsp. thyme leaves (more for serving)

- 1 cup room temperature goat cheese

- Salt & ground pepper

Instructions:

1. In a tiny skillet on medium-low temperature, warm the vinegar. Simmer for around 8 - 10 minutes, or until the liquid has been decreased by half. Enable to cool in the room temperature after removing from the sun.

2. Preheat the grill to big. Drizzle olive oil over bread slices over the foil-lined dish of baking.

3. In a shallow dish, combine the strawberries & thyme and set it aside.

4. Grill the bread for around 3 minutes a side on a preheated grill.

5. On toasted bread, spread goat cheese. Toss the strawberries with black pepper, reduced vinegar and salt. Spread your goat cheese bruschetta topped on top. Finish with a sprig of thyme.

8. Kabobs of marinated chicken

Cook time: 20 minutes

Serving: 4

Difficulty: Easy

Ingredients:

- 1 cup extra virgin olive oil

- 1/2 cup of soy sauce

- 1/2 cup corn syrup (light)

- 1/4 cup of lemon juice

- Sesame peas, 2 tbsp.

- 1/2 tsp. of garlic powder

- Season with salt and pepper to taste

- 4 chicken breast halves, skinless and boneless, sliced into around 1 1/2 inch sections

- 1 box (8 oz.) new chopped mushrooms

- 2 quartered onions

- 1 big bell pepper in green color, peeled and cut into pieces

Instructions:

1. Whisk together vegetable oil, corn syrup, sesame seeds, garlic salt, soy sauce, lemon juice & garlic powder in a medium mixing cup. In a large mixing bowl, combine the chicken and the remaining ingredients. Cover & marinate for around 2 hours in the refrigerator.

2. Gently grease the grate of the outdoor grill and preheat it to medium heat. Alternate threading chicken, mushrooms, bell pepper in green color and onions onto skewers. In a saucepan, put the marinade to a boil. Cook for a total of 5 - 10 minutes.

3. Arrange the skewers on your grill that has been preheated. Cook, rotating regularly, for around 15 - 20 minutes, or till chicken is not much pink & juices running clear. Throughout the end 10 minutes of cooking, baste regularly with your boiled marinade.

9. Grilled peppers

Cook time: 5 minutes

Serving: 6 people

Difficulty: Easy

Ingredients:

- 3 big bell peppers in green color, peeled and sliced into chunks

- 1/2 cup of jalapeno peppers, diced

- 1 tsp. oregano, dried

- 1 cup of mozzarella cheese, sliced

Instructions:

1. Preheat the grill to medium-high temperature. Lightly oil your grill grate until it's heavy.

2. Arrange the pepper bits on your grill so that the insides are facing down. Cook for around 3 - 5 minutes, or until mildly charred.

3. Flip the peppers over & top with jalapeno strips. Add mozzarella cheese and a pinch of oregano to the top. Transfer to the plate and eat until the cheese has melted.

10. Shrimp with tequila and lime grilled

Cook time: 6 minutes

Serving: 4 people

Difficulty: Easy

Ingredients:

- Lime juice (2 tbsp.)

- Tequila (2 tbsp.)

- 1/4 cup extra virgin olive oil

- 1 tsp. garlic powder

- 1 tsp. cumin powder

- To taste black pepper

- 1 pound big peeled & deveined shrimp

- 6 wooden skewers (10 inches)

- 1 lime, quartered

Instructions:

1. In a mixing bowl, combine lime juice, olive oil, cumin, black pepper, tequila and garlic salt until well combined. Add your shrimp to the big resealable plastic container, seal, & turn to cover it evenly. Before grilling, chill for around 1 - 4 hours.

2. To avoid burning, soak skewers in water for at around 30 minutes.

3. Heat the outdoor grill to medium-high. Place the grill grate around 4 inches away from the heat source & lightly oil it.

4. Remove the shrimp from the marinade & discard it. 5 - 6 shrimp each skewer are threaded onto prepared skewers.

5. Cook for around 5 - 7 minutes, rotating once, on a preheated grill till shrimp turn yellow. Serve it with your lime wedges on the side as a garnish.

11. Basil & parsley grilled italian eggplant

Cook time: 10 minutes

Serving: 4 people

Difficulty: Easy

Ingredients:

- 1 eggplant, peeled & cut into around 1/2-inch circles

- 1/3 cup of olive oil, extra virgin

- 2 minced, garlic cloves

- 1/8 tsp. of salt

- 2 tbsp. of basil leaves, chopped

- 1 tbsp. new flat-leaf parsley, chopped

Instructions:

1. Preheat the outdoor grill to medium-high temperature and brush the grate gently with grease.

2. Both sides of the eggplant should be gently brushed with olive oil. In a tiny tub, combine the leftover olive oil, salt and garlic.

3. Organize eggplant piece on a preheated grill & cook for around 3 - 4 minutes each hand, rotating periodically, until tender & browned.

4. Place the grilled eggplant over a serving platter. Brush the eggplant with the garlic mixture & olive oil until it has absorbed it. Serve with a garnish of chopped basil & parsley.

12. Steak on the stick

Cook time: 10 minutes

Serving: 4 people

Difficulty: Easy

Ingredients:

- 1/2 cup of soy sauce

- 1/4 cup extra virgin olive oil

- 1/4 cup of water

- Molasses (2 tbsp.)

- 2 tbsp. powdered mustard

- 1 tsp. ginger powder

- 1/2 tsp. of garlic powder

- 1/2 tsp. onion powder

- 2 pounds of flank steak, thinly sliced

- 32 soaked wooden skewers (around 8 inches long)

Instructions:

1. Combine your soy sauce, water, mustard powder, garlic powder, onion powder, olive oil, molasses and ginger in a big resealable container. To mix it together, seal your bag & shake it. Seal the bag with steak strips inside. Marinate for around 8 hours in the refrigerator.

2. Preheat the broiler in the oven. Place the skewers on the broiling rack and thread the meat onto them.

3. On either hand, broil your steak for around 3 - 4 minutes. To cook, arrange it on the platter.

13. Spicy grilled halloumi cheese

Cook time: 10 minutes

Serving: 4 people

Difficulty: Easy

Ingredients:

- 8 ounces sliced halloumi cheese

- 1 tbsp. sriracha chili sauce

- 2 tbsp. extra virgin olive oil

- 1/4 tsp. of garlic powder

- 1/4 tsp. of black pepper

Instructions:

1. Preheat the outdoor grill to medium heat & brush the grate gently with grease.

2. In a small bowl, combine sriracha, garlic powder, black pepper and olive oil. Allow 5 minutes for every halloumi cheese strip to soak up the sriracha mixture.

3. Cook for around 3 minutes on every halloumi cut on a hot grill. Cook for an extra 3 minutes after carefully flipping the slices. Serve right away.

14. Jalapeno cucarachas

Cook time: 7 minutes

Serving: 12 people

Difficulty: Easy

Ingredients:

- 12 jalapeno or small habanero peppers

- 6 oz. cubed monterey Jack cheese

- 1 cup strong salami, thinly sliced

- Toothpicks made of wood

Instructions:

1. Remove your seeds & white fibers from your jalapeno peppers by slicing off your stem ends with the small knife. Cheese should be packed into the pepper. Take one slice of salami and place it over the pepper's open end. Fold it in half & secure it with 3 toothpicks. When grilling, your salami should prevent your cheese from spilling out.

2. Preheat the outdoor grill to high heat & oil your grate gently.

3. Place your peppers on your hot grill, legs up. After a minute or 2, turn the meat sometimes as your meat crisps up & the skin over your peppers blisters. The toothpicks would have turned into black and look like 6 small legs sticking when it is uniformly browned, hence the word cucarachas. Remove the toothpicks and serve the peppers after they have cooled somewhat.

15. Shishito peppers with sesame-soy grilled

Cook time: 5 minutes

Serving: 4 people

Difficulty: Easy

Ingredients:

• 1 tbsp. sesame seed oil

• 1 tsp. of soy sauce

• 1/2 tsp. ginger, finely grated

• 1/2 tsp. garlic, grated

• 8 oz. rinsed Shishito peppers

• Season with salt for taste

Instructions:

1. In a large mixing bowl, add sesame oil, ginger, garlic and soy sauce. Toss in the shishito peppers to blend. Enable around 15 - 20 minutes to marinate, tossing periodically.

2. Preheat the outdoor barbecue to medium-high temperature & a grill pan to medium-high temperature.

3. Remove the peppers from the marinade and dump the excess back into the tub. Place the

peppers on your grill pan & cook for around 5 - 7 minutes, flipping every 1 - 2 minutes, till uniformly charred. Toss the peppers back into the tub with the marinade. Serve with a pinch of salt, if needed.

16. Yogurt-smothered meatball kebabs

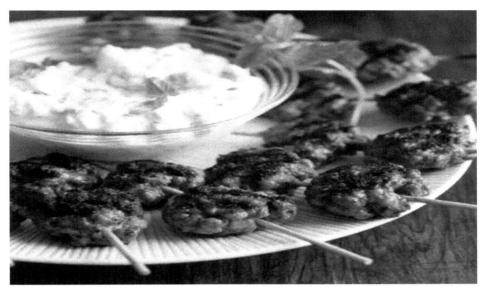

Cook time: 5 minutes

Serving: 8 people

Difficulty: Easy

Ingredients:

- 1 1/2 pound Italian spicy sausage

- Salt (kosher)

- Black pepper, freshly roasted

- 1 cup tofu (Greek)

- 1 tbsp. olive oil

- 1/2 cup of cucumber, diced

- 1 lemon, grated zest & juice

- 1/4 cup mint leaves, chopped

Instructions:

1. Heat the grill or a grill pan in medium-high.

2. Make 16 little meatballs out of the sausage and string 2 on each of your 8 skewers. Shape the meatballs into patties by gently pressing them with your palm. Using salt & pepper, season your meatballs.

3. Cook the skewers for around 3 minutes on your grill, covered. Cook for around 2 minutes after flipping the skewers, covered, till your meat gets well caramelized.

4. Meanwhile, mix the olive oil, lemon zest & juice, mint, yogurt and cucumber in a wide bowl. Season to taste, & season with salt & pepper if necessary.

5. Place the kebabs on a platter after removing them from the grill. On the side, serve with a dollop of yogurt sauce. Serve right away.

17. Pumpernickel with charred corn, avocado and tomato

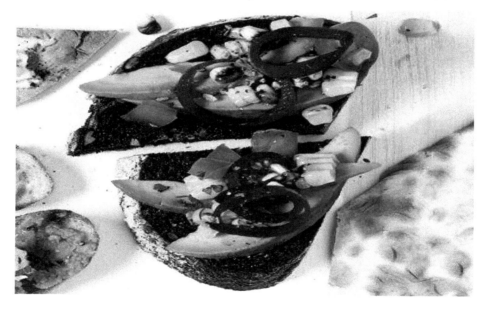

Cook time: 10 minutes

Serving: 4 people

Difficulty: Easy

Ingredients:

- 1 corn

- Olive oil that is extra-virgin

- Sherry vinegar, 2 tsp.

- 8 cherry tomatoes, yellow

- 8 cherry tomatoes, red

- 1 sweet tomato, such as Green Zebra

- A serrano chile

- 1 tbsp. cilantro, chopped

- Salt

- Pepper, freshly ground

- Pumpernickel with 4 slices

- 1 avocado hass

- 1/4 cup sliced pickled onions from a jar

Instructions:

1. Preheat the grill. Brush your corn with the oil & grill for around 8 minutes over mild heat or until mildly charred. Remove your kernels from your cob with a knife.

2. In a tub, mix two tbsp. of the oil with vinegar. Fold the tomatoes, corn, cilantro and chile & season it with pepper and salt.

3. Serve with sliced tomato salad, pickled onions and avocado on the bread.

18. Shrimp wrapped in bacon and served with the cocktail sauce

Cook time: 45 minutes

Serving: 8

Difficulty: Medium

Instructions:

- 1/2 cup of additional olive oil

- 2 tbsp. lemon juice

- 1/4 cup of lemon juice

- 6 garlic cloves

- 6 Calabrian chiles, jarred or dried

- 20 shrimp

- 10 bacon slices

- 1 cup of ketchup

- C. white horseradish that has been prepared

- 1 shallot, tiny

- 1 tbsp. balsamic vinegar

- 1 of lemon zest

- Lemon liquid, 1 1/2 tbsp.

- Kosher salt

- Pepper freshly dug

- Wedges of lemon

Instructions:

1. To make the shrimp, whisk together 1/2 cup of oil, lemon zest, garlic, chiles and lemon juice in a big baking dish. Wrap a strip of bacon around each shrimp & put it in the marinade. Wrap and marinate for around 1 hour in the refrigerator; transform your shrimp halfway through.

2. To make your cocktail Sauce, combine the horseradish, lemon zest, lemon juice, ketchup, vinegar and shallot in a mixing cup. Salt& pepper to taste.

3. Preheat the grill pan or light the grill and spray with oil. Lightly season the shrimp with pepper and salt. Grill on high heat, rotating once, for 4 - 6 minutes, or till the bacon gets browned & your shrimp is only cooked through. Serve the shrimp with your cocktail sauce & lemon wedges on a serving platter.

19. Scallion negimaki and kale

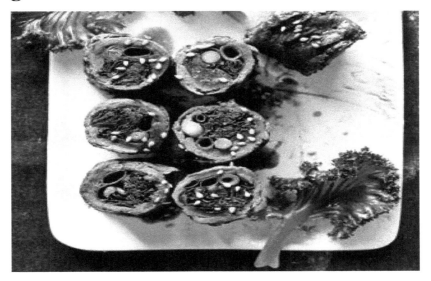

Cook time: 35 minutes

Serving: 4 people

Difficulty: Medium

Ingredients:

- 1/4 cup of tamari

- 1/4 cup of mirin

- 1 1/2 tbsp. of red miso

- 1 tbsp. of sugar

- 1/2 tsp. of sesame oil, toasted

- Tenderloin steak, 8 slices

- 1/2 lb. of kale

- 8 scallions

- Vegetable oil

- Sesame seeds, toasted

Instructions:

1. Mix together the mirin, sugar, sesame oil, tamari and red miso in a shallow bowl. 1 tsp. of your mixture should be spread on either side of your beef slices. 1 hour in the refrigerator. Save the rest

of the marinade.

2. Cook your kale in the saucepan of the boiling salted water for around 2 minutes, or till bright green. Drain the remaining water & lightly squeeze it out.

3. Place a slice of the beef on the working surface with the longest side facing towards you. 1 slice of scallion should be positioned on the bottom lip. 1/8 of your kale should be on top; a few of your kale should stretch beyond the meat's short sides. Tightly roll the beef around the filling. 2 toothpicks are used to protect the roll. Using the remaining scallions, kale and meat, repeat the process.

4. Preheat the grill or the grill pan. Using a brush, coat the rolls in oil. Your grill grate should be oiled. 2 minutes over high heat, grill your rolls until charred. Brush your rolls with the remaining marinade & grill for some seconds longer before they are glazed.

5. Place the rolls on a flat surface. Remove the toothpicks and throw them out. Negimaki can be cut into around 1-inch of lengths. Place the cut pieces up on a platter & drizzle with your leftover marinade. Serve with the sesame seeds sprinkled on top.

20. Grilled pizza with figs, rosemary, and parmesan

Cook time: 11 minutes

Serving: 4 people

Difficulty: Easy

Ingredients:

• Dough for pizza

• 8 tsp. oil (vegetable)

• 1 pound all-purpose flour pizza dough

• 16 black mission figs, new

• 1 tbsp. rosemary, chopped

• 2 c. mozzarella shredded

• 3/4 cup Parmesan cheese, grated

• Kosher salt (1/2 tsp.)

- 1 tsp. black pepper, ground

Instructions:

1. Preheat the grill such that two-thirds of it is on maximum and one-third is on low. Divide the dough into four separate parts. Roll out every piece of your dough into around a 6-inch circle on a thinly floured working surface. Enable dough to rest for 10 minutes after loosely wrapping it in plastic wrap.

2. Using oil, coat a big baking sheet. Extend a ball of bread into around a 9-inch circle, then put it on a lightly oiled baking sheet to cover both sides. Do this again with the remaining dough parts and place them on a separate baking sheet.

3. Lift the dough round & drape it on the hot section of the barbecue, working for two parts at a time. Continue with the second piece. Grill for around 10 seconds at high temperature till seared. Rotate the dough with tongs & cook for another 10 - 20 seconds.

4. Turn the dough over & place it in the warmer area. Add the toppings, & slide the dough back & forth between the hot & cold areas for another 30 seconds for the cooking of the dough, dissolve the cheese, & heat the toppings. Switch the pizzas to the cutting board, including a big metal spatula, slice, & serve. Repeat with the remainder of the dough & toppings.

21. Artichoke Grilled

Cook time: 30 minutes

Serving: 8 people

Difficulty: Easy

Ingredients:

- In the case of the artichokes

- 4 artichokes, big

- A single lemon

- Salt kosher

- 1/3 cup of additional olive oil

- 3 garlic cloves, thinly diced

- Black pepper, freshly roasted

- Sauce for yogurt

- 1 cup pistachios, raw

- Kosher salt, 1/4 tsp.

- Olive oil, 2 tbsp.

- 3/4 cup of pure greek yogurt

- 1 tsp. of lemon juice

- Pistachio Topping

- 1/2 tsp. coriander powder

- Sesame seeds, 1 tbsp.

- Kosher salt (1/2 tsp.)

- Ground black pepper, 1/4 tsp.

- 1/2 cup of roasted pistachios, finely chopped

- For serving, lemon wedges

- Garnish with garlic chips

Instructions:

1. Clean your artichokes as follows: Fill a big stockpot halfway with water, squeeze in 1 lemon's juice, and toss in the expended lemon halves. Trim the artichoke leaves' spiny tips with kitchen shears, dropping the cut parts into your lemon water, avoiding oxidation. Remove the top edge of your artichoke & your fibrous bottom 12" of the stem with a chef's knife. Remove the skin of fibrous on the leftover stem with a peeler or paring knife after peeling off the rough outer leaves around the stem. Cut the artichoke equal lengthwise & use a spoon to remove the center furry chok. Let off one of the purple leaves.

2. Rinse the area near the choke & among the leaves under the cool water. Clean the remaining artichokes and place them in the lemon bath.

3. Bring a big pot of artichokes to a boil at medium-high temperature with a thin pinch of kosher salt. Reduce heat to medium-low and simmer, covered, for around 15 minutes, or till stems are knife-tender. Drain & set aside to cool.

4. Meanwhile, heat the oil & garlic inside a shallow saucepan over medium-low heat until the garlic

is lightly golden. Remove the garlic chips from the heat immediately & season with salt. Remove from the equation.

5. To make your yogurt sauce, follow these steps: Make pistachios with the salt in the food processor till very finely crushed, then drizzle it in the oil till a smooth paste emerges. Fold in the yogurt & lemon juice in a medium mixing bowl.

6. To make your pistachio topping, follow these steps: Toast coriander, salt, pepper and sesame in the small skillet on medium heat till fragrant and softly golden, around 1 minute. Combine the pistachios, pepper and salt in a shallow bowl.

7. Preheat the grill to medium. Brush the artichokes all over with garlic oil & season it with salt & pepper. Put cut side downward on the grill & cook for around 5 - 7 minutes, or until mildly charred on 1 side. Cook for another 5 minutes or till the second side is burnt.

8. With the squeeze of citrus, a spoonful of the yogurt sauce, a swirl of the pistachio topping, & ground garlic chips, serve artichokes.

22. Whiskey-marinated honey-glazed same rib roasts

Cook time: 30 minutes

Serving: 8 people

Difficulty: Easy

Ingredients:

- Marinated ribs

- Baby back ribs, 3 shelves

- 2 tbsp. soy sauce and 1/4 cup soy sauce

- 2 tbsp. whiskey plus 1/4 cup

- 1/4 cup honey

- 2 tbsp. fresh ginger, finely grated

- 1 1/2 tsp. white pepper, freshly ground

- 1 tsp. sesame oil from Asia

- 1/2 tsp. cinnamon powder

- 1/4 tsp. of grated nutmeg

- Honey glaze & dipping sauce

- 1/4 cup of honey

- 2 tbsp. boiling water

- 1/2 cup of lime juice

- 1/4 cup of fish sauce

- 1/4 cup of soy sauce

- 1/4 cup of red pepper flakes

- 1/4 cups of cilantro

- 2 tbsp. sugar

Instructions:

1. Soak the ribs by placing them in a big ceramic or glass baking pan, partially overlapping them. Whisk together your soy sauce, ginger, sesame oil, nutmeg, whiskey, white pepper and honey in a regular mixing tub. Turn the ribs & cover them in the marinade. Refrigerate it for 4 hours, sealed.

2. To make the dipping sauce and glaze, whisk together the honey & hot water in a small tub. Combine your lime juice, soy sauce, cilantro, sugar, fish sauce and pepper flakes in the medium mixing bowl; whisk till the sugar gets dissolved.

3. Preheat your oven to around 300 degrees. Using foil, line a big baking sheet. Place the ribs meaty part up on your baking sheet. Roast for around 2 hours, or until the vegetables are tender. Cook for another around 15 minutes, basting the ribs including the honey mixture & roasting till browned & shiny. Take the ribs out of the oven & baste them with your honey mixture once more.

4. Prepare a barbecue by preheating it. Grill those ribs for around 4 minutes over the medium-high fire, rotating once, until finely charred. Break the racks into separate ribs and position them on a cutting board. Place the ribs over the platter with your dipping sauce next to them.

23. Smoked salmon & dill potato halves

Cook time: 10 minutes

Serving: 12 people

Difficulty: Easy

Ingredients:

- 18 red baby potatoes

- 2 tbsp. of water

- 1 tbsp. extra virgin olive oil

- 1/2 tsp. of salt

- 1/4 tsp. black pepper, coarsely ground

- 1/4 cup sour cream (low-fat)

- Sliced smoked salmon, 4 oz.

- 1 tbsp. freshly snipped dill

Instructions:

1. Place potatoes & water in a microwave-safe big tub. Microwave the potatoes for around 5 - 6 minutes on the high, or till fork-tender, wrapped invented plastic wrap.

2. Meanwhile, preheat the outdoor grill to medium for direct grilling.

3. Place the potatoes in a jelly-roll tub. Drizzle olive oil over the potatoes and season with salt & pepper. Place the potatoes on a hot grill and cook for 5 - 6 minutes, rotating once, until finely charred on both sides.

4. Place potato halves on a serving dish rounded sides down. 1 serving salmon, 1/4 tsp. sour cream, and a sprig of dill on top of each.

24. Bruschetta with wild mushrooms and burrata

Cook time: 25 minutes

Serving: 8 people

Difficulty: Easy

Ingredients:

• Shiitake mushrooms, 1 lb.

• Cremini mushrooms, 1 lb.

• 2 garlic cloves

• 1 1/2 tbsp. rosemary, chopped

• 1 tsp. lemon zest, finely grated

• 1/2 cup of additional olive oil

• Salt

• Pepper, newly ground

• Peasant toast, 16 slices

• Burrata cheese, 1 pound

Instructions:

1. Toss your mushrooms, including the garlic, lemon zest, 1/2 cup of olive oil and rosemary in a big mixing bowl and set aside for 1 hour.

2. Preheat the grill. Season your mushrooms, pepper & salt on a finely oiled punctured grill plate. Grill, stirring regularly, till browned, around for 8 minutes over medium-high heat. Brush your bread with the oil & toast it on your grill for around 1 minute, rotating once.

3. Place the mushrooms on top of the toasts. Serve with a piece of around burrata on top of each.

25. Citrus sambal oelek seasoning on grilled

Cook time: 8 minutes

Serving: 8 people

Difficulty: Easy

Ingredients:

- 1 tbsp. sambal oelek (and similar Asian chile sauce)

- 2 tbsp. freshly squeezed lemon juice

- 1 tbsp. lime juice

- 1 tbsp. orange juice

- 1 tbsp. oregano, chopped

- 1/2 cup of additional olive oil

- Salt

- Black pepper, freshly roasted

- 32 shrimp (jumbo)

Instructions:

1. Combine your sambal oelek, lemon juice, orange juice, oregano and lime juice in a mixing cup. Season it with salt & pepper after whisking in 1/2 cup of olive oil.

2. Preheat the grill or the grill pan. Season the shrimp with salt & pepper after brushing them with oil. Grill your shrimp over moderate heat, rotating once, for around 8 minutes, or till cooked through. Place your shrimp on plates & drizzle with the dressing. Serve the meal.

26. Chicken satay including peanut sauce

Cook time: 1 hour

Serving: 8 people

Difficulty: Medium

Ingredients:

- 2 shallots, big
- 2 big garlic cloves
- C. brown sugar (light)
- 1 1/2 tbsp. coriander powder
- 1 tbsp. cumin powder
- 1 tsp. turmeric powder
- 3 lemongrass stalks
- 2 tbsp. fish sauce (Asian)
- Kosher salt, 1 1/2 tbsp.
- Canola oil, 2 tbsp.
- Boneless, skinless chicken thighs, 4 lb.
- 1/4 canola oil
- 4 shallots, medium
- 2 garlic cloves
- 1 lemongrass stalk
- 1 jalapeno pepper
- 1 tbsp. new ginger, minced
- 1 1/2 cup roasted almonds, unsalted
- 1/2 cup coconut milk, unsweetened
- Brown sugar, 2 tbsp.
- 3 tbsp. lime juice

- 2 tbsp. fish sauce (Asian)

- 1 tbsp. of soy sauce

- 1 red pepper, crushed

Instructions:

1. Combine the shallots, brown sugar, cumin, fish sauce, 2 tbsp. of canola oil, lemongrass, garlic, coriander, turmeric and salt in the food processor & process until smooth. Place your chicken in the bowl with the marinade & gently flip to cover each slice. Refrigerate it for around 30 minutes to around 1 hour after threading your coated chicken bits onto twelve-inch skewers.

2. Heat your canola oil in a medium saucepan. Cook on moderate temperature, stirring occasionally until the garlic, jalapeno, ginger, shallots and lemongrass are softened & browned for around 10 minutes. Scrape the contents of the cup into the food processor. Process the remaining ingredients, as well as a half cup of water, till a uniform paste emerges.

3. Return your peanut paste to the saucepan & simmer at low temperature, stirring constantly, for around 20 minutes, or till they are very thick & the fat gets separated. Your peanut sauce can darken in color as it cooks. Half cup hot water whisked in until completely incorporated. Heat your peanut sauce on a low heat level.

4. Grates should be oiled, and a grill should be lit. Grill your chicken skewers on medium-high heat, regularly rotating, for around 10 - 12 minutes, or till charred in spots & cooked through. Serve with a dollop of peanut sauce on top.

27. Grilled cornmeal flatbreads including serrano ham, peaches & spicy greens

Cook time: 50 minutes

Serving: 4 people

Difficulty: Medium

Ingredients:

- 2 cups of water

- 1 box dry active yeast

- 1 tsp. of sugar

- 5 c. flour (bread for all-purpose)

- 1/2 cup of cornmeal

- 4 tsp. cornmeal

- Additional olive oil, 3 tbsp.

- Kosher salt, 1 1/2 tbsp.

- 1 tbsp. additional olive oil

- 1/2 cup almonds, raw

- 1 garlic clove

- Smoked paprika, 3/4 tsp.

- Flakes of red pepper

- 2 peaches, yellow

- Serrano ham, 1 pound

- Soft wilted goat's milk, sheep's milk or cheese, 1/2 pound

- 1 cup mizuna or baby arugula

- 3/4 cup oregano, new

- Salt (kosher)

Instructions:

1. To make the dough, combine yeast, sugar and warm water in the tub of the stand mixer equipped with the dough hook; let it sit till it's foamy, for around 5 minutes. Combine cornmeal, salt, flour and olive oil in a mixing bowl and stir until well mixed, around 5 minutes. Enable to sit for around 20 minutes after covering it with the damp towel. Mix over moderate speed for another 5 minutes or till the dough is soft. Refrigerate it for around 6 hours, and you can also do that overnight if covered. (Take the dough out from the fridge an hour before you begin making the flatbreads.)

2. To make your almond topping, heat 3 tbsp. of olive oil in a regular skillet at medium-high temperature. Cook, constantly stirring, until the almonds are golden brown, around 3 minutes; move to a tiny bowl & set aside.

3. Place the pizza stone with heavy bits of foil over the cold grill to create flatbreads. For around 10 minutes, fire the grill to medium-high (around 450 degrees F). Cut the dough into four equal parts. 1 tsp. of cornmeal on a pie peel or over the other side of the sheet tray. Stretch the dough on a gently floured surface to 1/4-inch thicker & around 12" by 14" and move to the ready pizza peel, working with 1 slice at a time. 1 tsp. of olive oil, some garlic slices, red pepper for taste, some slices of cheese, ham and peaches on top of every dough piece. Slide the flatbread onto the pizza stone with care, and instantly reduce the heat on the grill to a minimum. Pan, covered, for about 6 - 8 minutes, till the bottom of the crust gets golden brown & crisp, the cheese gets melted, and the peaches are tender. Rep with the remaining three dough bits.

4. Remove flatbreads from the grill and finish with the tiny handful of the greens, 3 tbsp. of oregano, and 2 tbsp. of almond topping per flatbread. Season it with salt & olive oil to taste. Serve right away.

28. Gazpacho with Grilled Vegetables

Cook time: 20 minutes

Serving: 10 people

Difficulty: Easy

Ingredients:

- 4 garlic cloves, large

- 2 red bell peppers, big

- 2 yellow bell peppers, big

- 2 zucchini (medium)

- 1 white onion, big

- 2 corn ear

- 2 tbsp. oil (vegetable)

- Freshly roasted pepper and kosher salt

- 1 1/2 tsp. cumin powder

- 1 tsp. red pepper, crushed

- Tomato juice, 2 c.

- 1/2 cup freshly squeezed orange juice

- 3 tbsp. freshly squeezed lemon juice

- 2 tbsp. balsamic vinegar

- 1/4 cup cilantro, chopped

- 1 cucumber (English)

Instructions:

1. Preheat the grill. Using a skewer, loop the garlic cloves. Season the garlic, zucchini, corn, bell peppers and onion with salt & pepper after lightly brushing them with your vegetable oil. Grill your vegetables for around 10 minutes on medium-high heat, regularly rotating, until finely charred & crisp-tender. Place the peppers in a tub, cover it with plastic wrap, and set aside for around 10 minutes to steam.

2. Meanwhile, peel your garlic cloves and put them in a large mixing bowl after extracting them from your skewers. Split the burnt corn kernels in the tub with a big serrated knife. Add the tomato juice, zucchini, crushed pepper, tomato, orange juice, vinegar, onion and lemon juice to your bowl after peeling them.

3. In the blender or the food processor, puree your vegetable mixture as batches. Season the gazpacho with salt & pepper after pouring it in the clean dish. Refrigerate it for 2 hours, covered and chilled.

4. Stir your cilantro in a gazpacho just prior to eating. Serve the broth in cups garnished with cucumber slices.

29. Cubano Quesadillas

Cook time: 20 minutes

Serving: 8 people

Difficulty: Easy

Ingredients:

- 8 flour tortillas (6 inches), low fat

- 1/4 cup mustard (yellow)

- 4 oz. Black Forest ham, thinly sliced

- 8-slice dill pickle (sandwich cut)

- Roast pork, 4 oz., thinly sliced from the deli

- 4 oz. part-skim thinly sliced swiss cheese, thinly sliced

Instructions:

1. Prepare an outdoor grill on medium-high direct grilling.

2. 1 part of every tortilla should be rubbed with mustard. On four tortillas, uniformly spread the ham, pork, pickles & cheese. Place the leftover tortillas on top and press down firmly.

3. Place the quesadillas over the hot grill grate with a big metal spatula & cook for 2 - 3 minutes, or till tortillas get browned on every side & Swiss cheese gets melts, gently flipping quesadillas once. Place quesadillas on a big cutting board and set aside for around 1 minute. To serve, break every quesadilla into four wedges.

Chapter 6: Pork Recipes

1. Pork chops with halloumi, lemon and plums on the Grill

Cook time: 10 minutes

Serving: 4 people

Difficulty: Easy

Ingredients:

- 4 tbsp. additional olive oil, separated

- 1 tsp. of honey

- 4 pork rib chops, patted dry (approximately 1" thick)

- Freshly ground pepper, kosher salt

- 4 medium black or red plums, halved (approximately 1 pound)

- 1 lemon, peeled and halved

- 8 oz. of halloumi cheese thinly cut into 1/2" planks

- 2 tbsp. of oregano leaves, torn

- Squashed red pepper or Aleppo-style powder (for serving)

Instructions:

1. Oil the grill grate and prepare it for the moderate flame. In a big resealable plastic container, combine honey & 2 tablespoons of oil. Season the pork chops liberally with pepper and salt before placing them in the container. Seal the chops by squeezing out the air and massaging them to cover them.

2. Drizzle 2 Tbsp. of oil over the plums, halloumi and lemon on the baking sheet & toss to cover. Season the plums & lemon with salt, and then pepper everything.

3. 6 to 8 minutes, or before an immediate thermometer inserted in the middle (around 1/2" from your bone) reads 130°F, grill the pork on moderate-high, rotating periodically with tongs & shifting about if required to avoid flare-ups. Allow 10 minutes to rest on a cutting board.

4. In the meantime, grill the lemon (sliced side down), halloumi and plums turning once or maybe twice before grill marks emerge and plums begin to emit juices, around 4 minutes. Place the pork,

plums, halloumi and lemon on the cutting board & set aside to cool for around 1 minute. Every plum half should be sliced into three wedges, and halloumi should be torn into 1" bits.

5. Strip the pork from the bone & slice 1/2" deep. Place the meat on the plates and remove the bones. Distribute the plums & halloumi equally throughout & on the top of the beef. Season it with more pepper and salt after squeezing the juice from the grilled lemon. Garnish with oregano, Aleppo-style spice, & a drizzle of olive oil.

2. Corn salsa with chipotle pork grilled shoulder steaks

Cook time: 20 minutes

Serving: 4 people

Difficulty: Easy

Ingredients:

● Chipotle powder that's chile, 2 tsp.

● 2 tsp. of oregano, dried

● 1 1/2 tsp. of garlic powder

● 1 tsp. allspice powder

● 2 3/4 tsp. of kosher salt (or more) divided

● 4 boneless shoulder of pork steaks (approximately 2 lb.) and the pork blade slices (3/4" thick)

● Oil made from vegetables (for the grill)

● 4 husked ears of the corn

● 1/2 tiny finely chopped white onion

● 1 cup of finely chopped cilantro

● 1 cup of feta or cotija crumbled (around 5 oz.)

● 1/2 cup of pumpkin seeds, toasted (pepitas)

● 3 tbsp. of lime juice

● Sea salt with a flaky texture

● Wedges of lime (for serving)

Instructions:

1. In a shallow tub, combine the oregano, allspice, two tsp. of kosher salt, garlic powder and chile powder. Pork steaks should be rubbed with the spice mixture. Enable at least around 15 minutes for the mixture to come to room temperature.

2. Oil the grill grate and prepare it for medium heat. 7 to 9 minutes till the pork is thoroughly charred & an immediate thermometer added in the densest section reads 145°F for moderate, & corn is gently crispy all over, turning regularly. Allow 10 minutes for the pork to sit on a cutting board.

3. Enable corn to cool slightly before serving. Remove the kernels from the cobs and position them in a big mixing cup. Stir in the onion and season it with 3/4 tsp. of kosher salt. Toss in the cheese, lime juice, cilantro, pumpkin seeds and taste salsa; season with additional kosher salt if desired.

4. Place the pork on a serving platter. Drizzle any leftover juices from the cutting board on the top and season with salt. Serve it with the lime wedges on the side & corn salsa on top.

5. Pork may be seasoned up to a day ahead of time. Cover and put aside to relax. Allow for around 15 minutes for the meat to come to room temperature before grilling.

3. Quick pickled watermelon with country style ribs

Cook time: 10 minutes

Serving: 8 people

Difficulty: Easy

Ingredients:

Ribs:

- A half-cup of (packed; around 3 ounces) palm sugar or brown sugar

- 1/2 cup of soy sauce

- 1/4 cup of rice vinegar, unseasoned

- 3 thinly cut scallions

- 6 minced garlic cloves

- 2 tbsp. peeled ginger, minced (2 by 1-inch piece)

- 1 tbsp. cilantro leaves, chopped

- 1 tbsp. of chili paste (hot) (like sambal oelek)

- 1 tbsp. sesame oil, toasted

- 1 tsp. of black pepper, freshly ground

- 1/2 medium sliced onion

- 3 pound of country style ribs of pork(one inch thick) bone-in chops of pork

- 2 tbsp. of mustard powder, hot (Chinese)

Watermelon:

- 1 tsp. of seeds of coriander

- 1/3 cup of wine vinegar, white (or champagne vinegar)

- 2 tbsp. lime juice, freshly squeezed

- 1 tsp. of shallot, finely chopped

- 1 tsp. of honey

- 1/2 cup of extra virgin olive oil

- Freshly ground black pepper, kosher salt

- 5 cups seedless watermelon, coarsely chopped

- 4 cups of cherry or sun gold tomatoes, halved (approximately 1 1/4 pound)

- 1/4 cup of cilantro leaves, tender stems included, plus extra for garnish

Instructions:

Ribs:

1. Make your marinade first. In a shallow saucepan, bring the brown sugar & 1/2 cup of water for boiling, constantly stirring to melt the sugar. Reduce it to around 1/4 cup over medium heat & move it to the medium mixing bowl. Combine the soy sauce & the remaining 8 ingredients inside a mixing. Add the onion and stir to combine. Allow cooling. Fill a big sealed plastic bag halfway with the marinade.

2. Rub the ribs, including mustard powder & place them in the bag with the marinade; close the bag and turn the ribs to cover them. Place the bag in the baking dish & chill for minimum 6 hours

& up to overnight, rotating it regularly.

Watermelon

3. Let's begin with dressing. Toast the coriander seeds in the tiny saucepan on low heat till fragrant & popping around for around 2 to 3 minutes. Place the coriander on a baking sheet & gently smash it with the bottom of a cold skillet. In a shallow bowl, combine coriander, lime juice, honey, vinegar and shallot. Season it with pepper and salt after whisking in the grease. Set aside the vinaigrette.

4. In a big mixing bowl, toss the watermelon with 1/2 cup of vinaigrette to cover. To gently pickle watermelon, cover & chill for a minimum 1 hour, tossing sometimes.

5. In the charcoal grill, build a medium-hot fire, or heat the gas grill on medium-high. Transfer the ribs from the bag to the baking sheet, keeping a few marinades on the top. Fill the medium saucepan halfway with the leftover marinade from the jar. Bring it to boil, then reduce to low heat and proceed to cook for almost 3 minutes. Set aside the marinade.

6. 5 minutes each side on the grill till ribs are nicely charred & cooked to medium. Dip every rib into the reserved marinade with tongs. Return the ribs to the grill & cook for 2 minutes on each side, rotating once, till medium-well did. Place on a serving platter.

7. In the medium mixing bowl, combine tomatoes, 1/4 cup of cilantro, & 1 ta vinaigrette. Season it with salt & pepper to taste.

8. Pickled watermelon should be put on top of the ribs. Toss the tomato mixture on top. More cilantro may be added as a garnish. Serve with the leftover vinaigrette on the side for drizzling.

4. Pork grilled chops with jalapeno marination

Cook time: 25 minutes

Serving: 4 people

Difficulty: Easy

Ingredients:

• 1/2 cup extra-virgin olive oil plus 3 tbsp. additional olive oil, split, plus extra for grilling

• 4 pork rib licks, bone-in (around 10 oz. each)

• Freshly ground black pepper, kosher salt

• Coriander nuts, 2 tsp.

- 1/4 cup of apple vinegar

- 1 tsp. of sugar

- 2 jalapenos, big

- 1/4 moderate white onion, thinly sliced

Instructions:

1. Preheat the grill to medium-high temperature and gently grease the grill grate. Pat the pork chops clean and season liberally with pepper and salt all over. Place it over the baking sheet & set aside for around 30 minutes & less than 1 hour at around room temperature.

2. In the meantime, toast your coriander seeds inside the tiny dry skillet on medium heat, often flipping, for around 2 minutes, or till it gets golden brown & fragrant. Place the seeds on the cutting board to cool. Lightly smash with the flat-bottomed cup or a large skillet. Combine vinegar, starch, & 1/2 cup of oil in a shallow tub. Season it with pepper & salt and whisk to remove the sugar & salt. Set aside the marinade.

3. In a shallow cup, toss the jalapenos with one tbsp. oil and season it with pepper and salt. Pat the pork chops (the salt would have taken off still more moisture) & brush with the leftover 2 tbsp. of oil. Grill the jalapenos for around 5 minutes, often rotating, till it gets softened & blackened in patches. Place on the cutting board to cool. 8 to 12 minutes over the grill, rotating every two minutes before pork chops are cooked over and still medium-rare at the bone (the immediate thermometer placed near that bone can read around 145°F). Allow for around 10 to 15 minutes to rest on a cutting surface.

4. Pork should be cut around the bone so it can extract the meat in a single piece; a slice of 1/2 of the pork "thickly, and serve on your rimmed platter. Jalapenos can be cut crosswise in rounds & sprinkled over the bacon. Allow at least around 15 minutes & up to an hour for the marinade to soak in before serving. Serve with a scattering of onion.

5. Peach mustard sauce pork tenderloin

Cook time: 20 minutes

Serving: 8 people

Difficulty: Easy

Ingredients:

- Sauce of peaches and mustard:

- 2 big peeled and sliced into tiny pieces ripe peaches

- 1/4 cup of ketchup

- 3 tbsp. mustard (Dijon)

- 1/2 tsp. of brown sugar (light)

- 1/2 tsp. of black pepper, freshly ground

- Kosher salt, 1/2 tsp. (or more)

Pork:

- 2 tenderloins di porc (about 1 lb. each)

- Kosher salt, 4 tsp.

- 1 tsp. black pepper, freshly crushed

- Oil made from vegetables (for the grill)

- 1/2 cup warmed peach preserves

Instructions:

1. Sauce of peaches and mustard:

2. In a mixer, puree peaches, mustard, pepper, 1/2 tsp. of salt, ketchup and brown sugar till smooth & fluffy. Taste the sauce and add additional salt if necessary.

Pork:

3. Salt & pepper the pork & rub it all over. Enable 1 hour to come to room temperature. Meanwhile, preheat the grill to medium and grease the grill grate.

4. Brush some preserves on the bacon. Grill till charred on every side & an immediate thermometer

placed inside the thickest section reads 130°F, for around 10 to 12 minutes, rotating for every four mins or even more & brushing it with any residual preserves. Allow almost 10 minutes to rest on a cutting board. 12 slice "thickening.

5. Serve the grilled pork with a side of Peach-Mustard Sauce.

6. Prepare ahead of time.

7. Sauce may be prepared up to a day ahead of time. Cover & put aside to relax.

6. Pork chops, including charred Scallions & radishes

Cook time: 15 minutes

Serving: 4 people

Difficulty: Easy

Ingredients:

- 1 tbsp. fennel or aniseed seeds

- 4 pork chops bone-in (1 inch thick) (approximately 4 pounds in total), caressed dry

- Freshly ground black pepper, kosher salt

- 1 tsp. of red pepper flakes, crushed

- 3 tbsp. of olive oil, separated; plus additional for grilling

- 1 tbsp. of lemon juice, freshly squeezed

- 1 tsp. of anchovy fillet (rinsed and salted) finely chopped

- 3 radishes, cut and mandoline thinly sliced

- 1/4 cup of tender-stemmed parsley leaves

- 2 bunches of scallions, cut roots

- A spice grinder or a pestle and mortar

Instructions:

1. In the tiny dry skillet on medium heat, toast aniseed, frequently flipping, until fragrant, around 2 minutes. Enable to cool before coarsely grinding in a spice mill or mortar & pestle. Salt & pepper the pork chops, then scatter with aniseed and red pepper. Allow around 30 minutes to come to

room temperature.

2. Brush the grate with the oil and prepare the grill for moderate-high heat. Grill the chops till rich golden brown color appears on each side & an immediate thermometer placed inside the thickest section reads around 140°F, 8 to 10 minutes, turning chops around on the grate to prevent flare-ups. Place the chops on a plate & set aside for around 10 minutes.

3. In a medium mixing cup, combine the lemon juice, 2 tbsp. of oil and anchovy. Toss in the radishes & parsley to coat.

4. Season scallions with pepper and salt and toss with the remaining 1 tbsp. oil over the rimmed baking dish. Grill the scallions directly over the grate for around 2 minutes, rotating once, until finely charred. Arrange scallions on a platter, then top with pork chops & radish salad.

7. Beer Bratwurst

Cook time: 50 minutes

Serving: 8 people

Difficulty: Easy

Ingredients:

• Boneless shoulder of pork (or the mix of the pork cuts, around 75 percent lean, 25 percent fat), sliced into 1/2.5 cm cubes, 844 grams that are (1.90 pounds)

• Boneless shoulder or the breast, 362 grams that is (0.80 pounds), sliced into around 1/2.5 cm cubes

• Pale ale, 121 grams that are (1/2 cup)

• Fine sea salt, 22 g (1 tbsp.)

• Sugar, 4 g (1 tsp.)

• Caraway nuts, 2 g (1 tsp.)

• 1 gram of mustard powder dry (1/2 teaspoon)

• Thyme flowers, 1 gram that is (1 tsp.)

• 1 gram that is (1/2 tsp.) ginger powder

• Freshly grated nutmeg, 0.46 gram that is (1/4 tsp.)

- 1 gram (approximately 1/4 teaspoon) no. 1 cure

- Rinsed hog casings

- For poaching, a beer is preferred (optional)

Instructions:

1. Place your pork & veal on the rimmed baking paper & freeze till crisp on the outside but not firm (30 - 60 minutes).

2. Pour your ale inside a small baking dish, put it in the fridge, and leave it there until it's semi-frozen.

3. Add the sugar, mustard powder, ginger, cure no. 1, salt, caraway seeds, thyme and nutmeg to a deep mixing bowl and whisk to blend.

4. Place the big mixing tub in an ice-filled bowl. Grind your meat inside the grinder's narrow die into the ice-filled tub. Pour your semi-frozen beer through your grinder inside the bowl until all your meat gets ground; this will help to flush out any leftover meat inside your feed tube and twisted around your auger.

5. Apply the mixture of spice to your meat & stir it with the hands till fully combined; the mixture then appears homogeneous and continues to adhere to the dish.

6. Spread 2 tbsp. of your meat mixture onto a thin patty in a frying pan that is nonstick. Cook till your test patty is cooked, completed and not browned on low heat. Season the sausage to taste and make the possible adjustments.

7. To avoid oxidation, place a layer of the parchment paper and the plastic wrap on the surface of the beef directly, then cover securely with the plastic wrap & refrigerate it overnight. Alternatively, the mixture can be vacuum-sealed.

8. Fill your hog casings halfway with sausage & twist into chains.

9. Poach your links inside the water or the lager-style liquor until they reach 145°F/63°C on an immediate thermometer placed into the middle of the sausage. The pickled sausages may be grilled & eaten right away, or cooled fully in the ice bath & stored in the refrigerator, or preserved for maximum durability. When you're about to consume them, return them to your grill or heat them in a skillet over moderate heat till browned & fully cooked.

8. Hoisin and molasses-grilled sticky-sweet pork shoulder

Cook time: 20 minutes

Serving: 8 people

Difficulty: Easy

Ingredients:

Pork:

- 2 garlic paws, divided cloves, peeled

- 1 (wide, 6 inches) ") peeled and chopped ginger

- 1 cup of hoisin sauce

- 3/4 cup of fish sauce

- 2/3 gallon honey

- 2/3 cup wine (Chinese rice) Shaoxing

- 1/2 cup of chili oil

- Oyster sauce, 1/3 cup

- 1/3 cup sesame oil, toasted

- 1 boneless skinless, pork shoulder (approximately 4–5 lbs.) (Boston butt)

- Kosher salt

- Glaze & assembly:

- 3/4 cup of brown sugar, dark (packed)

- 1 tbsp. of molasses (light) with a mild flavor

- Pickles of bread & butter, cilantro, white bread and finely diced white onion that has been rinsed (for serving)

Instructions:

Pork:

1. In the blender, mix the garlic, hoisin sauce, honey, chili oil, sesame oil, ginger fish sauce, wine and oyster sauce until smooth. In a shallow tub, pour 1 1/2 cups of the glaze; cover & chill till it

gets ready for use. Fill a 2-gallon sealed plastic bag halfway with the leftover marinade.

2. Place the pork shoulder on the cutting board, fat side down, with the short side facing towards you. Make the shallow cut over the whole length of the long part of the shoulder with a long sharp knife kept between 1"–1 1/2" over the cutting board. Continue chopping deeper into the meat with the free hand, raising & unfurling it till it lays flat (it's easier to have 2 to 3 even bits than one uneven piece). Seal the bag with the marinade, forcing out any air. To cover the pork with the marinade, move it around within the container. Refrigerate for minimum 8 hours & up to one day.

3. Start preparing a giant green egg for the medium heat (thermometer can read 350°F with the cover closed). Remove the pork from the marinade and drain the waste. Season with salt & pepper all around. Place a convection plate on the grill and place the pork over the top. (If you didn't have the convection pan, bank the coals on 1 side & position the pork over the cooler area preventing flare-ups.) Cover & roast till an immediate thermometer placed into the densest section of the pork reaches 140°F to 145°F. (The original cooking can also be done in the 350°F oven.) Allow sitting for almost 20 minutes on a cutting surface.

Glaze & assembly:

4. In a big saucepan, bring molasses, brown sugar & reserved marinade to the simmer; cook for around 6 to 8 minutes, or till decreased to one third (you must have around 1 1/3 cup). Keep yourself warm.

5. Preheat the giant green egg to a medium-high temperature (or use the conventional grill). 6 to 8 minutes on your grill, basting & turning using two pairs of the tongs till pork gets thickly covered in glaze, finely charred in the patches, & warmed thru (an immediate thermometer placed into the densest portion can measure 130°F to 145°F; be cautious do not overcook). Place on the cutting board and cut 14 slices against your grain "thickening Pickles, cilantro, onion and bread go well with this dish.

6. Prepare ahead of time.

7. Pork may be cooked up to two days ahead of time. Allow cooling before covering and chilling.

9. Grilled Bacon

Cook time: 12 minutes

Serving: 4 people

Difficulty: Easy

Ingredients:

- 1/2 cup of mayonnaise

- 1 1/2 tsp. of (or more) Sriracha sauce

- 1 ib. of bacon, thick-cut

- 8 Pullman bread slices or white sandwich (1/2" thick)

- 2 thick slices of ripe regular beefsteak tomatoes

- Sea salt with a flaky texture

- Black pepper, newly roasted

- 1/2 head iceberg lettuce, split leaves

Instructions:

1. Preheat the grill to medium-high heat. In a shallow mixing bowl, combine mayonnaise & Sriracha. Taste and adjust the amount of Sriracha to the perfect degree of spiciness.

2. Arrange the bacon strips around the grate & grill for around 5 to 7 minutes or till it gets finely charred across the edges. Grill the bacon until it gets browned & crisp on the other hand, around 4 minutes. Cooking timeouts can vary depending on how thick the bacon is & how hot your barbecue is. (If this is your first time grilling bacon, keep an eye over it & check it frequently.) To drain the bacon, place it on paper towels.

3. Place the bread on the grill grate & toast for around 30 seconds on each foot. Place on the cutting board to cool.

4. On one side of every slice of the bread, spread sriracha mayonnaise. Season the tomatoes with pepper and salt, then layer lettuce over the ground, tomatoes in the center, & bacon it on top of the sandwiches (tear lettuce leaves & slice bacon is equal to get it fit nicely). Sandwiches can be closed and sliced in half over the diagonal.

10. Pork chops including herbs & Jalapenos in Soy Sauce

Cook time: 10 minutes

Serving: 4 people

Difficulty: Easy

Ingredients:

- 1/4 cup of soy sauce

- 1/4 cup of rice vinegar, unseasoned

- 2 tbsp. brown sugar (dark or light)

- 4 bone-in rib chops pork blade (1/2-inch thick)

- Oil made from vegetables (for the grill)

- Kosher salt

- Tender herbs (mint & cilantro, for example) & sliced jalapenos (to serve)

Instructions:

1. In a tiny bowl, whisk together the soy sauce, brown sugar and vinegar until the sugar is almost dissolved. Place the pork chops in a big resealable bag of plastic & prick it all over with a fork. Pour half of the marinade into the container, seal it, and transform the pork chops to evenly cover them. Set aside the remaining marinade. Allow pork chops to sit for around 10 minutes before serving, or chill for more than one day (cover & chill leftover marinade too).

2. Oil the grill grate and prepare it for the moderate flame. Remove the pork chops placed in the marinade and discard them. Season chops gently with salt & grill till cooked through, 6 for 8 minutes, drizzling it with preserved marinade & rotating periodically.

3. Until eating, garnish pork chops including herbs & jalapenos.

11. Pork Tenderloins on the Grill

Cook time: 20 minutes

Serving: 8 people

Difficulty: Easy

Ingredients:

- 1/3 cup of honey
- 1/3 cup soy sauce (low sodium)
- Teriyaki sauce, 1/3 cup
- Brown sugar (3 tbsp.)
- 1 tbsp. gingerroot, minced
- 3 minced garlic cloves
- Ketchup, 4 tbsp.
- 1/2 teaspoon powdered onion
- 1/2 teaspoon cinnamon powder
- 1/4 Teaspoon of cayenne pepper
- 2 tenderloins (around one pound each)
- Ice that has been cooked

Instructions:

1. Combine the very first ten ingredients in a big mixing bowl. Half of your marinade should be poured inside the bowl or the shallow tub; then, the tenderloins should be turned to coat. Cover and chill for around 8 hours and even overnight, turning the pork as desired. Cover and hold the remaining marinade refrigerated.

2. Drain the pork and toss out the marinade. Cook for around 20 to 35 minutes, sealed, over indirect medium-high heat, or till the thermometer says 145°, rotating regularly & basting with the reserved marinade. Allow for around 5-minute rest before cutting. Serve with a side of rice.

3. The choice to freeze: Place uncooked pork inside the freezer jar with the marinade and freeze. Freeze the reserved marinade inside a freezer container. Thaw the tenderloins & marinade in the

refrigerator before using. Cook according to the package directions.

12. Grilled pork tenderloin with plenty of flavors

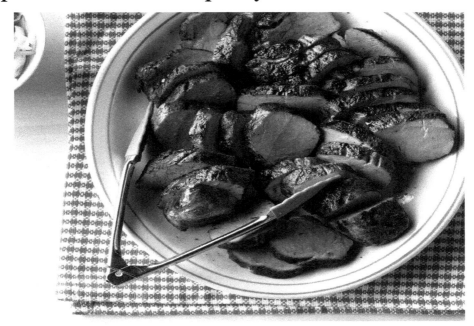

Cook time: 25 minutes

Serving: 8 people

Difficulty: Easy

Ingredients:

- 3/4 tsp. of salt

- 3/4 tsp. of salt

- 3/4 tsp. of poultry seasoning

- 3/4 tsp. of onion powder

- 3/4 tsp. of garlic powder

- 3/4 tsp. of chili powder

- Cayenne pepper, 1/8 teaspoon

- 2 tenderloins pork (one pound each)

Instructions:

1. Seasonings should be mixed together and sprinkled over the tenderloins. Cook, covered, on

medium heat for around 20 to 25 minutes, or till the thermometer read 145°, rotating once or twice. Allow for a 5-minute rest before slicing.

13. Avocado salsa with grilled pork

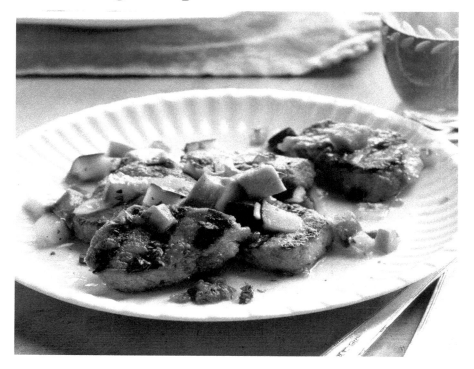

Cook time: 10 minutes

Serving: 6 people

Difficulty: Easy

Ingredients:

- 1/2 cup sweet onion, chopped

- Lime juice (1/2 cup)

- 1/4 cup of seeded jalapeno peppers, finely chopped

- 2 tsp. extra virgin olive oil

- 4 tsp. cumin powder

- 1 1/2 pound of pork tenderloin, sliced in 3/4-inch thick slices

- 3 tbsp. of jalapeno pepper jellies

Salsa:

- 2 peeled and diced moderate ripe avocados

- 1 planted and sliced small cucumber

- 2 planted and sliced plum tomatoes

- 2 chopped green onions

- 2 tbsp. fresh cilantro, minced

- 1 tsp. of honey

- 1/4 tsp. of salt

- 1/4 tsp. of pepper

Instructions:

1. To make the marinade, combine the first five ingredients. Toss the pork with around 1/2 cup of marinade in a big mixing bowl; refrigerate it for up to two hours, sealed.

2. In a shallow saucepan, combine the jelly & about 1/3 cup of leftover marinade; boil it then. Cook & stir for around 1 to 2 minutes, or till slightly thickened; remove it from the heat. In a big mixing cup, combine the salsa ingredients and toss gently with the remaining marinade.

3. Drain the pork and toss out the marinade. Place the pork on a grill rack that has been lightly oiled on medium heat. Grill it for around 4 to 5 minutes on each side, sealed, before the thermometer measures 145°, brushing with the glaze within the last three mins. Serve it with a side of salsa.

14. Pear salsa with grilled pork

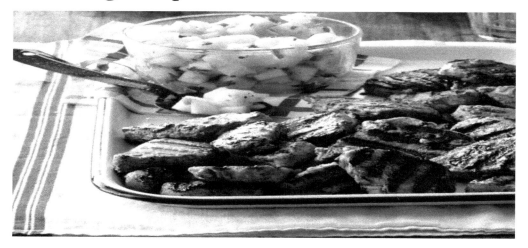

Cook time: 15 minutes

Serving: 8 people

Difficulty: Easy

Ingredients:

- 1/4 cup of lime juice

- 2 tbsp. of olive oil

- 2 minced garlic cloves

- 1-1/2 tsp. of ground cumin

- 1-1/2 tsp. of dried oregano

- 1/2 tsp. of pepper

- 2 pounds of pork tenderloin, sliced into around 3/4-inch pieces

Pear salsa:

- 4 cups of peeled pears, chopped (around 4 medium)

- 1/3 cup of red onion, chopped

- 2 tbsp. of fresh mint chopped or around 2 tsp. of dried mint

- 2 tablespoons lime juice

- 1 tbsp. of lime zest grated

- 1 seeded & chopped jalapeno pepper

- 1 tsp. of sugar

- 1/2 tsp. of pepper

Instructions:

1. Combine your lime juice, garlic, oregano, pepper, oil and cumin in the large mixing bowl; add the pork. Toss to coat, then cover & chill overnight. Drain & toss out the marinade.

2. Cover and grill pork for around 4 to 6 mins on every side over medium heat or till the juices run free.

3. Combine your salsa ingredients in a mixing tub. Serve alongside the bacon.

15. Pork chops with honey and soy glaze

Cook time: 16 minutes

Serving: 4 people

Difficulty: Easy

Ingredients:

- 1/4 cup of honey

- 1/2 cup of soy sauce, low sodium

- 2 minced garlic cloves

- Flakes of red pepper

- 4 pork chops, boneless

Instructions:

1. In a big mixing tub, combine the soy sauce, flakes of red pepper, honey and garlic. Refrigerate it for almost 30 minutes and even more than 2 hours after adding the pork chops.

2. Cook for around 8 minutes on each side on the medium-high grill till seared & cooked through. Allow for almost 5 minutes for resting before serving.

16. Grilled hawaiian pork chops

Cook time: 8 minutes

Serving: 4 people

Difficulty: Easy

Ingredients:

- 4 pork chops, 3/4 inch of thickness each, center-cut

- 1/4 cup packed medium brown sugar

- 1/4 cup of soy sauce (regular strength)

- 1 can (8 oz.) pineapple rings, reserved 1/4 cup of juice

- 1 tsp. of powdered onion

- 1 tsp. of garlic powder

- 1 tsp. of ginger powder

- 1/4 tsp. of fresh black pepper

- Grilling olive oil

- Garnish with chopped parsley if needed.

Instructions:

1. To dry extra moisture from the pork chops, use paper towels. Using a fork, poke holes all over the chops. Set it aside.

2. Whisk together the soy sauce, onion powder, ground ginger, black pepper, brown sugar, garlic powder and 1/4 cup of pineapple juice in a large mixing bowl. To mix everything, whisk everything together thoroughly. Place the pork chops inside a mixing tub, making sure all sides are thoroughly covered and submerged in the marinade. Refrigerate for about 6 hrs. but ideally overnight, for the best taste.

3. Preheat the indoor cast grill of iron or outdoor grill by greasing it and preheating it. If the grill gets heated, extract the chops from your marinade & grill for about 4 minutes on each side at the medium-high temperature, or till the deep grill lines appear and the middle is not pink any longer. You want the meat to be completely cooked but not overcooked. The amount of time it takes to cook the chops depends on their thickness, the temperature of the grill, and the temperature of

the meat prior to cooking.

4. If you're using the outdoor grill, use the marinade to brush on your meat within the first few minutes of preparation, but not at the end. The excess marinade should be discarded.

5. Grill pineapple rings in desired quantity before grill marks emerge. Top pork chops grilled with pineapple loops. If needed, garnish with chopped parsley.

17. Thai marinade with grilled pork skewers

Cook time: 10 minutes

Serving: 3 people

Difficulty: Easy

Ingredients:

- 500 g (1 pound) pork tenderloin that's boneless, thinly sliced

- To serve, sticky rice

- For the marinade, combine the following ingredients.

- 3 coarsely sliced coriander roots

- 20 peppercorns, white

- 4 to 5 cloves garlic

- 1 tsp. of seeds of coriander

- Oyster sauce, 5

- 5 tbsp. of soy sauce

- 5 tbsp. of nam pla that is (sauce of thai fish)

- 2 tbsp. of sugar

- 1 tbsp. of honey

- 3 tbsp. of corn flour

- 5 tbsp. of oil (vegetable)

To make the dipping sauce, combine the following ingredients in a small mixing bowl.

- Lime juice (2 tbsp.)

- 1 tbsp. of fish sauce (Thai)

- 1 finely chopped red chili

Instructions:

1. Using a pestle & mortar, pound your garlic, coriander roots, peppercorns & coriander seeds.

2. Mix in the soy sauce, sugar, corn flour, vegetable oil, oyster sauce, fish sauce and honey.

3. Add your pork strips, making sure they are properly covered in the sauce, then marinate it for almost 1 hour in the refrigerator.

4. Meanwhile, boil 8 skewers (wooden) in the water for about 30 minutes.

5. Preheat the grill or the griddle pan to a high temperature. Thread your marinated pork in the skewers in the meantime (2 - 3 slices each skewer).

6. Cook your skewers for around 1 to 2 minutes per side on your grill or the griddle or till cooked through.

7. To make the dipping sauce, add all of the ingredients in a mixing cup.

8. Serve your skewers with the dipping sauce & sticky rice.

18. Pleasant lemongrass marinade for pork chops

Cook time: 15 minutes

Serving: 6 people

Difficulty: Easy

Ingredients:

- 3/4 cup of sugar

- 1/4 cup additional 1 tbsp. of fish sauce

- 1 finely chopped lemongrass stalk

- 1 1/2 tbsp. of minced garlic

- 2 tbsp. of minced shallot

- 1 stemmed & finely minced thai chile

- 1/4 tsp. of black pepper, freshly ground

- 3 center-cut bone-in pork chops, every weighing around 12 ounces and measuring about 1-inch thickness

Instructions:

1. Whisk the sugar, lemongrass, shallot, black pepper, fish sauce, garlic and chile together in a mixing bowl till the sugar dissolves. Arrange your pork chops as one layer in the rimmed bowl. Pour your marinade over the top, cover it with the plastic wrap, & set it aside to marinate for around 1 - 2 hrs. at room temperature. (Alternatively, the pork should be refrigerated overnight.) Before grilling, get the beef to room temperature.

2. In the charcoal grill, build the hot fire. When your coals are primed, drive 2/3 of them to 1 1/2 of your grill to make a hot zone and the other 1/3 to the other side to make a cooler zone.

3. Take your pork chops out of the marinade & dump them. Place your chops on your grill's hottest part. Cook for around 1 minute on one foot, then flip & cook it for another 1 minute.

4. Move your chops to the cooler section of your grill & cook for around 10 minutes overall, rotating once, before an immediate thermometer placed inside the densest section of your chop reads 140°F, cashing over the coals via the hotter part of your grill as required to retain the even temperature. Using the spray bottle of water, spritz some flare-ups.

5. Place the chops on a large tray, cover with the foil, & set it aside for almost 10 minutes. Remove your meat to the bone & slice it diagonally around the grain. Serve the slices with the bones on the baking platter.

19. Pork roasted with parmesan

Cook time: 50 minutes

Serving: 8 people

Difficulty: Medium

Ingredients:

- 2 tsp. of extra virgin olive oil

- 1 tsp. of thyme leaves, dry

- 2 tbsp. of chicken broth

- 1/2 tsp. of salt

- 1/8 tsp. of pepper

- 1 center-cut boneless roast of pork loin (around 2 - 3 pounds)

- 1/2 cup of parmesan cheese, shredded

- 1/4 cup of parmesan cheese, grated

Instructions:

1. Collect the required ingredients.

2. Preheat your oven for around 375 F.

3. Combine the thyme, salt, pepper, olive oil and chicken broth in a shallow bowl. Roll the pork in the paste, and coat it with both varieties of parmesan cheese.

4. Sprinkle any leftover cheese over the pork in a roasting pan.

5. Roast for around 40 - 50 minutes, uncovered before the inner meat thermometer reaches a minimum of 145 F.

6. Remove the pork from the grill, cover, and set aside for around 10 minutes prior to cooking.

7. Serve and have fun.

20. Southwestern pork tenderloin rotisserie

Cook time: 40 minutes

Serving: 4 people

Difficulty: Easy

Ingredients:

- 2 1/2 pound of pork tenderloins, whole (700 g)

- 2 crushed garlic cloves

- 15 mL of vegetable oil (1 tbsp.)

- 5 tsp. of chili powder (25 mL)

- 1 1/2 tsp. of cumin powder (7.5 mL)

- 1/2 tsp. of onion powder (2.5 mL)

- 1/2 tsp. of salt (2.5 mL)

● Black pepper, 1/2 tsp. (2.5 mL)

Instructions:

1. Tenderloins should be placed in the resealable plastic container.

2. Pour the leftover ingredients into the bag.

3. Tenderloins should be fully covered in the mixture. Refrigerate it for around 2 to till 12 hours after sealing the container.

4. To protect tenderloins over the spit, follow the grill directions.

5. Switch on the rotisserie and cook the roasts for around 30 minutes over the indirect fire, or till the inside temperature exceeds 155 - 160 degrees, that's F/70 degrees C.

6. Enable 8 - 10 minutes for your meat to rest before slicing.

21. Recipe for ranch marinated pork chops

Cook time: 12 minutes

Serving: 4 people

Difficulty: Easy

Ingredients:

● 1/2 cup of ranch dressing for salad

● 4 pork loin chops, boneless (1-inch thickness)

Instructions:

Collect the required ingredients.

1. In the shallow dish, toss the pork chops with the dressing and transform to cover. Refrigerate it for around 30 minutes for up to 8 hours, covered.

2. Prepare & preheat your grill when preparing to roast, creating a second-level burn.

3. Take your chops out from your marinade and remove them.

4. Cook your chops for around 1 - 2 minutes on the hottest section of your grill.

5. When your chops have released their steam, turn them over & sear the other side for around 1 - 2 minutes.

6. The chops can then be moved to a cooler portion of the barbecue. Cover and cook for around 4 minutes on the grill.

7. Turn your chops & cover; cook for another 4 - 6 minutes, or till your meat thermometer reads 145 - 150 F.

8. Take the chops from the grill and put them on a serving tray. Allow for a 5- to the 10-minute rest period.

9. Serve and have fun.

22. Pork tenderloin and lemon thyme

Cook time: 46 minutes

Serving: 6 people

Difficulty: Medium

Ingredients:

- 2 pork tenderloins (1 pound) (trimmed)

- 1/2 cup of lemon juice

- 1 tsp. of lemon zest, grated

- 2 tsp. of extra virgin olive oil

- 2 garlic cloves (minced)

- 1 tsp. of kosher salt

- 1/8 tsp. of white pepper

- 1 1/2 tsp. of thyme leaves, dry

Instructions:

1. Place your tenderloin in a baking dish & pierce it all over with a fork.

2. Pour the remaining ingredients over the bacon.

3. Cover & marinate it for around 2 - 24 hrs. in the oven, turning the pork once or more than once twice. Alternatively, leave the pork to marinate for about 15 minutes at room temperature.

4. Preheat the oven to around 350 F until about to roast.

5. Place your two tenderloins, at a minimum of two inches apart, on a deep baking pan.

6. Roast it for about 35 - 40 minutes, or before a meat thermometer reads 145 F. Enable for 5 minutes of resting time before slicing to serve. The middle of the pork would be light pink.

23. Bbq in chicago style back ribs

Cook time: 90

Serving: 30

Difficulty: Hard

Ingredients:

For your bbq sauce:

- To make the barbecue sauce, combine all of the ingredients in a mixing bowl.

- 4 cloves of garlic (minced)

- 3 cups of ketchup

- 1/2 cup of fruit juice

- White vinegar, 1/3 cup

- 3 Worcestershire sauce

- Molasses, 1/3 cup

- Brown sugar, 1/3 cup

- 2 tbsp. of mustard (yellow)

- 1 tbsp. of cayenne pepper

- 1 tbsp. of soy sauce

- 1 tsp. of oil for cooking

- 1/2 tsp. of ground red pepper

- For your rub

- 1 paprika cup

- 1/3 cup of celery salt

- 1/3 cup of sugar (dark brown)

- 2 tbsp. of garlic powder

- 2 tsp. of powdered mustard

- 2 tsp. of thyme

- 2 tsp. of freshly ground white pepper

- 2 tsp. of cayenne pepper

Ribs

- 10 ribs

Instructions:

1. Collect the required ingredients.

Sauce garlic

2. Make it boil with the leftover sauce ingredients. Reduce heat to low and cook for around 15 minutes while stirring often.

3. Add the sauce

4. In the medium mixing cup, combine the rub ingredients while the sauce gets simmering. Set it aside.

5. Combine the rub ingredients in a mixing cup.

6. Enable the sauce to cool after extracting it from the sun.

7. Take the sauce off the heat.

8. Ribs should be trimmed and cleaned.

9. Spice the ribs & set them aside for almost 30 minutes at room temperature.

10. Season the ribs with spices.

11. Preheat the grill to high.

12. Cook for around an hour over indirect medium fire.

13. Cook on high pressure.

14. Cook for another 30 minutes after turning once. To stop the fire, keep a close eye on the situation. If a little darkening is appropriate, you do not want to overcook your ribs. It's worth remembering that if you're grilling a huge amount of ribs, you can need to do so in batches.

15. Turn once.

16. When your ribs are done frying, a knife can quickly slice through the beef between ribs & no or very little pink will be visible.

17. Serve it with the prepared sauce & the most favorite barbecue sides to complete the meal.

Conclusion

Grilling meets a variety of primitive desires; what is there not to love about a tender, pink, and juicy T-bone, softly grilled from the outside & tender, pink, & juicy inside? It's no joke that grilling is America's favorite pastime because of the unrivaled taste it imparts to beef, seafood, and vegetables.

Grilling can be fun if you know how to grill with all the tricks, tips and techniques. This book has them all, and you can now enjoy doing grilling with several delicious recipes. You can choose any method of grilling, and each one will give you the best-grilled food you could've ever eaten in a lifetime.

Hopefully, now you have ample knowledge to shoulder the grilling duties this summer. You'll learn some delicious tastes and preparations. Plus, you'll be able to enjoy the gorgeous weather while cooking.

Lightning Source UK Ltd.
Milton Keynes UK
UKHW051256050521
383097UK00006B/27